# The Fit Body F.A.S.T. Method

The 4-Step Plan to Escape Weight Loss Traps, Burn Fat, & Stay Fit For Life—Without Wasting Your Time

Marcus Dennis

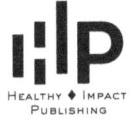

Healthy Impact Publishing

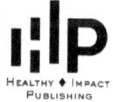

Healthy Impact Publishing

Charlotte, NC 28269

Copyright © 2025 by Marcus Dennis II

All rights reserved.

No portion of this book may be reproduced in any form without written permission from the publisher or author, except as permitted by U.S. copyright law.

This publication is designed to provide accurate and authoritative information in regard to the subject matter covered. While the publisher and author have used their best efforts in preparing this book, they make no representations or warranties with respect to the accuracy or completeness of the contents of this book and specifically disclaim any liability for any health and wellness-related outcomes that may occur as a result of applying the methods and/or principles found in this book. The information, advice and strategies contained herein may not be suitable for your specific situation, and therefore you should consult with a licensed health professional or practitioner when appropriate. Neither the publisher nor the author shall be liable for any loss of profit or any other commercial damages, including but not limited to special, incidental, consequential, personal, or other damages.

*Book Cover Design* by Marcus Dennis II

*Author Photo* by © Liz Golden

First Edition 2025

# Table of Contents

| | |
|---|---:|
| Disclaimer | VII |
| Before You Get Started... | 1 |
| Part I: The Four Principles Of A Fit Body | 10 |
| 1. The Seven Setbacks | 12 |
| 2. The Principle of Mindset | 30 |
| 3. The Principle of Function | 41 |
| 4. The Principle of Diet | 50 |
| 5. The Principle of Discipline | 68 |
| Part II: The F.A.S.T Method | 80 |
| 6. Focus | 82 |
| 7. Audit I: Boundaries & Accountability | 96 |
| 8. Audit II: Diet & Nutrition | 110 |
| 9. Strengthen | 128 |
| 10. Tweak | 234 |
| 11. Your Next Move... | 245 |
| Frequently Asked Questions | 247 |

| | |
|---|---|
| Acknowledgements | 252 |
| About the Author | 254 |

All glory to God.
For my wife and children, who inspire me every day to be a better husband, father, and coach.

# Disclaimer

This book, and the information contained herein, is intended for informational purposes only. It is not meant to disregard or act as a substitute for sound advice provided by a licensed medical or health professional. For your safety and well-being, please consult with your doctor concerning your health prior to starting any diet or exercise regimen.

# Before You Get Started...

"Every day is a chance to begin again. Don't focus on the failures of yesterday, start today with positive thoughts and expectations."
-Catherine Pulsifer

What if I told you that what you do in the next three months could determine the kind of body you'll have in the next three to five years? When it comes to burning fat, losing weight, and becoming fit, there's two things you should know: 1) it doesn't have to take as long as you think and 2) it's not as hard as you think to keep the weight off once you lose it. All you have to do is understand and recognize the patterns and principles that make weight loss predictable, then follow them.

Imagine for a moment that there was a fitness coach who had the ability to swap their mind with yours for twelve weeks. And within those twelve weeks, they would help you lose weight and whip you into the best shape of your life without you having to feel a thing. And imagine that with their knowledge, they would eat all the right foods, go through the pain of doing intense workouts, and adopt all the right habits to help you put your weight loss on autopilot. How do you think you would look and feel once you got your body back after those twelve weeks?

Let's take it a step further. Let's say that this coach handed you a checklist of everything they did to help you lose the weight and get in shape. What if, on this checklist, you saw that there were only *four* items you had to follow and the coach told you that if you did exactly what was on this list, then you would be able to keep the weight off for good? Would you follow the checklist to keep the results or go back to your old lifestyle and risk undoing everything?

## Is Your Fit Body a Focus or a Fad?

If you're like most people, you've probably tried a few diets, maybe had success with one or two of them and lost a fair amount of weight. But, after a few months, maybe a few vacations, or maybe after a few years, the weight eventually came right back. What's worse is that each time the weight came back, it took a heavier toll on your body more so than the previous time.

The reality is that you don't have as much time to work on your health goals as you think you do. According the the theory of changes in life phases, about every five or seven years or so, practically everyone will go through major life events or lifestyle changes. For example, usually five years after buying a new car, that's when your first major repairs tend to happen. If you have children, around every five to seven years they go through serious growth phases (i.e. early childhood to adolescence or adolescence to teenager, etc). Your body experiences this five to seven-year change as well. The body you had in your mid-twenties feels different than your early thirties and your body in your early thirties feel different when you reach your early forties, and so on.

You don't need me to tell you this because I know you feel it. You feel your body is getting older. Your job, whether it's more physical or psychological, has become more taxing and demanding on your body. You can't keep up with the kids or the grandchildren like you used to. You notice that certain activities that used to feel easy are now sapping your energy much quicker than normal. Here's the other thing: about 90% of people who go through a typical weight loss or lifestyle program, won't sustain their results past year five. The sad part is that every time this 5 to 7-year cycle happens, their body goes through another major change that makes it harder and harder to not only get results but keep them as well.

Most people treat their fitness goals and their body like a fad where it's fashionable and convenient to pursue during the summer season and the next season it's forgotten about. One moment, you're in the gym with a routine that's got you sweating your butt off and dropping pounds, and the next moment you're skipping workouts, binge-eating junk food, feeling stressed and depressed because the number on the scale isn't moving fast enough in the direction you wanted.

Before you know it, five years have gone by and you begin to question if you just wasted all of your time doing the wrong things. This may be something you've experienced in the past or maybe you're experiencing this right now. Either way, the more you treat your body like this, the longer you keep going through this cycle, the more it's costing you your results and the harder your fitness journey becomes in the future.

Do you think your body can handle another five years of new diets or weight loss programs? Are you ok with living in this cycle where your weight loss is a constant uphill battle as your body gets older or are you ready to make healthy living your focus?

## What Fit People Do and Why You Should Do It Too...

If you're ready to make being fit your focus, then there are two questions you might consider asking yourself that I believe just might change everything for you:

1) "What do the fittest and healthiest people do and how can I do more of that?"
2) "What do most people, who struggle with their health and weight loss do and how can I avoid doing that?"

I'll save you some time by telling you what fit people don't do. They don't follow the latest diet trends or fads, or take a laundry list of weight loss supplements, or spend hours at the gym doing Instagram workouts in order to stay lean and burn belly fat. I'm not against diet hacks, or supplementation, or flashy exercises, but these approaches generally don't work. Why? Because these are all popular methods that most people are doing in order to lose weight fast and it always works well for a while...until it doesn't.

That's not what this book is about.

## The Expectation

This book isn't about pushing a popular diet or promoting some revolutionary new workout regimen in order for you to get fit and lose weight fast. You won't find such strategies or methods in here. In fact, if you're looking for anything in this book that validates any of the popular beliefs, myths, or methods related to diet and weight loss, then this book is not for you.

The goal of this book is to *take you away* from doing what most people are doing, which is achieving short-term results by jumping from one cycle of failure and frustration to another, and give you the tools that health and fitness coaches *actually* use in order to get long-term results.

But how do you break the cycle? What separates those who can easily stay in shape and lose weight from those who constantly struggle with weight loss and fitness? Based on my experience, it seems to boil down to this:

**Most people, who struggle with their health and weight loss, look to follow a *process to fit their preferences* while those who are fit and healthy look to follow a *process to fit the principles.***

Just imagine how it would feel to...

- be comfortable and confident in your skin whether you're at work, in the gym, or on the beach.

- be able to eat and not worry about counting calories because the food you're eating *naturally* keeps you slim.

- be able to play your children or grandchildren without getting tired too easily or being able to pick them up without feeling weak.

- go to the gym or be physically active not because you *have* to, but because you *want* to.

- hear frequent compliments from your spouse about your physique because they notice the effort you're putting in week after week.

- wake up every morning and not have to think about stepping on a scale because you can see in the mirror that you're in the best shape of your life.

If any of those experiences sounded appealing to you, then I have good news: I wrote this book just for you! That 4-item checklist I mentioned earlier in that imaginary, mind-swapping scenario is based off of principles that I follow in order for me to stay in shape pretty much all-year round. With these principles, I was able to come up with a 4-step process that my clients and I could follow that would allow us to have access to those same experiences I just mentioned. And now, I'm sharing this process with you.

## Your Body, Your Results...

Now, as exciting as it would be for you to swap minds with a fitness coach for twelve weeks and have them do all the work for you, it's not the reality we live in. However, this book you're reading is the closest I can get to putting my brain, figuratively speaking, into your brain so that you can follow the same checklist that other health coaches and trainers like myself follow in order to get fit and stay in shape for as long as you want.

Of course results will vary, so please <u>DO NOT</u> compare yourself and the speed of your results with others. I don't know where your health and weight loss sit as priorities in your life nor do I know if you will take action and apply any of the material in this book. Therefore, I can't promise that you'll drop thirty pounds in three months or that you'll look and feel sexy by your next vacation. However, I *can* promise that if you keep doing the same things you've always done, then you'll keep getting the same results you've always had.

That being said, just reading the material won't do it for you. You still have to put in the work and go through this process, but once you do, you'll be free from the chaos and confusion that comes with the modern dieting and weight loss approaches and learn to take better control of your results, but more importantly your health. So, if that all sounds good to you, then let's get started! I'll see you in the next chapter.

For quick access to resources and additional guidance for the material, scan the QR code:

# PART I:

# THE FOUR PRINCIPLES OF A FIT BODY

"The man who grasps principles can successfully select his own methods. The man who tries methods, ignoring principles, is sure to have trouble."
                                        -Harrington Emerson

## Chapter One
# The Seven Setbacks

"The obstacle is the path."

-Sara Shepard

"If you don't learn from your experiences, you'll be destined to repeat them."

-Roy T. Bennett

It's Monday morning and you're at the office. You tell yourself, "No more excuses! This time, things will be different." You've planned out your meals, bought the groceries, even bought yourself that over-sized water bottle so you can stop slacking on your water intake. You finish with your last task of the day and rush off to the gym while you still have the time and motivation.

You make it to the gym parking lot, along with a hundred other cars that are all fighting for the closest spot to the entrance. After a few minutes of circling the lot with no success, you start to become irritable. Tiredness begins to set in and you feel your motivation dropping fast. You do your best to ignore how tired you are because you're still determined to get in shape and be healthy. Just then, a spot finally opens up and you pull right into the space without a second thought. You begin to feel a slight sense of relief because you finally made it to the gym!

You walk through the front doors, check in, and realize that the gym is obnoxiously crowded. After you get settled in, you make your way around the noisy gym atmosphere and scope out all of the machines.

You're a little nervous and overwhelmed at first, however you're still proud of yourself for taking that first step in keeping that commitment you made! Although you haven't fully thought about what body part you want to work on, you patiently wait to grab whatever machine becomes available. As soon as something opens up, you sit down, read the instructions, pick some random weight you feel is good to start with, then proceed to do as many repetitions as you can until you get tired.

You repeat this process at each machine a few more times and before you know it, an hour has passes by and you've just completed a full body workout. Mission accomplished! Now, all you have to do is keep up that momentum for the next few months. How hard can that be?

The first few days go great. After a couple weeks, you seem to be on a solid streak with your workout and dieting...until work explodes. Fires need to get put out, clients and customers need your help, the kids need some extra attention at home, your knees start to feel more crunchy than usual, and your old back pain flares up again. All of the sudden, you're skipping workouts, grabbing fast food, wondering how everything went downhill so fast, and asking yourself, *"what happened? Why is it hard to lose weight and stay consistent?"*

## Motivation & Willpower Are Not Always the Problem

You've probably told yourself that just need more willpower or more discipline. But what if I told you the real reason you keep falling short isn't a lack of motivation but rather it's the hidden roadblocks that are sabotaging your progress before you even start? They're the reason why 95% of weight-loss attempts fail within five years. These roadblocks aren't random...they're predictable.

In fact, there are seven of them that quietly control how quickly you get to see your results and how long you get to keep them. If you've ever wondered why almost every diet or workout plan you've ever tried eventually fails, this chapter is going to explain why...but more importantly, challenge you to take the next step in overcoming these obstacles.

## The Pitfalls

Out of the many hundreds, if not thousands, of conversations I've had with individuals who wanted to lose weight and make healthy lifestyle changes, the one question that I make sure to bring up in almost every conversation is, *"What's been holding you back?"* or *" What obstacles are in your way?".* What I've learned throughout my career by asking this question is that the people who struggle the most with weight loss and building long-term health habits, tend to fall into the same seven traps.

You may have experienced all of these at one point or maybe you can only relate to a few. In either case, if you can identify the problem then it's easier to come up with a solution. The first step is awareness, so here are the seven setbacks you need to watch out for that are keeping you stuck:

## 1. Poor Plan

There are only two kinds of plans that will affect your weight loss and fitness goals: a "good plan" and a "poor plan".

A good plan is a plan that looks at all angles and takes as many of your lifestyle factors as possible into consideration such as diet, environment, social interactions, resistance training, recovery, and more. A good plan tends to be predictable, looks farther into the future, and consists of both short-term and long-term goals. A good plan recognizes areas where you could fail but, more importantly, finds ways to make adjustments. A good plan follows health principles that allows you to customize your process in order to achieve a healthier lifestyle.

A poor plan does the opposite. It's short-sighted and mostly considers the results you can achieve as quickly as possible rather than the lifestyle to make those results last. A poor plan is usually unpredictable and deceptive because it can feel good to follow when things go right, but doesn't show you how to make adjustments when things go wrong. A poor plan has you copy other people's process and ignore health principles, which can lead to an unhealthy lifestyle.

The point here that when you don't have a specific, long-term plan for how you would like to achieve and sustain your weight loss, you set yourself up for long-term stress and frustration by default. The longer you continue to follow a plan or program that doesn't fit your desired lifestyle, even if you see *some* results, the more energy, time, and resources you lose. The short-term benefits will be inconsistent at best, which in turn will destroy your motivation for getting fit and eventually lead you to burnout.

That's why one of the first things new clients admit to me is that they don't have any idea where to start or what to do. They're tired of having short bursts of energy and motivation three months into their program only to fall off and start over three months later. If you don't know where to start or what to do, that's perfectly alright! It's better to be in a position where you're fully honest with yourself about not knowing what to do than to burn yourself out by cluelessly following a program that wasn't intentionally designed for you.

***Signs/Symptoms to Look For:***

- You frequently switch between diets or other programs

- You have no clear, structured plan on how to reach your initial weight loss goal

- Your plan is heavily influenced my social media trends or what "works for a friend"

- You're unsure of how to measure your progress beyond the scale

## 2. Inconsistency

One of the top reasons why people do not achieve their weight loss and fitness goals is because they struggle to be consistent. This is what most of my clients experience and it's usually the one they want to address as quickly as possible. Most people think they're inconsistent because they don't have a program to follow, when the truth is it's much more than that. Consistency requires discipline, and discipline works best when you have a clear goal and accountability.

Earlier, we outlined the importance of having a good plan or a clear goal and we'll soon discuss the impact of accountability. However, the point here is that as soon as you notice you're becoming inconsistent with your regimen, you open the door for things to go downhill pretty quickly.

Sometimes inconsistency can creep up on you simply because you haven't properly prioritized your health habits into your schedule or maybe you haven't thought to prioritize your health at all. It can be hard to have the motivation or discipline to create and stick with healthy habits if they aren't on the agenda ahead of time. The downward spiral of inconsistency can start with simple acts like waking up a little later in the morning because you didn't go to bed on time, going out of town due to a family emergency and forgetting to adjust your routine before you leave town, taking on that extra overtime instead going to the gym that afternoon like you had planned, and the list goes on.

If you don't find the time to prioritize your health habits then you essentially give others permission to set your priorities for you. There will always be things in life that happen and will throw you off track. There will most certainly be times where you don't feel like sticking to plan. The key is to still make your health habits a priority in your calendar. If you fall off track, reschedule that health-related task as quickly as possible and have an action plan in place to prevent interruptions as much as possible.

### *Signs/Symptoms to Look For:*

- You tend to start a program strong, but quickly lose momentum

- You frequently find reasons to skip workouts or seek convenient food options

- Your decisions to act on your program heavily depend on "feeling motivated"

- You find it hard to restart your program after you've fallen off

## 3. Tension

Tension is the state of mental unrest that throws you off balance physically and emotionally. Tension is stress, and it can be one of the reasons why you may be struggling with weight loss. If you're not properly managing your stress, you will have a very difficult time trying to reach your goal.

Cortisol is the hormone that comes to mind when you hear the word stress and it's often portrayed as the "bad hormone", however it's role in the body isn't bad at all. In reality, it's protective. Cortisol, the stress hormone, is responsible for helping you keep a circadian rhythm (i.e: your body's internal clock). In the morning, cortisol levels are generally at its highest because it allows your body to wake up, and when you go to sleep, those levels usually drop to its lowest. It's also responsible for your body's ability to metabolize glucose (blood sugar) so that your muscles have enough energy to respond to physical stress quickly during your "fight or flight" response.

The biggest problem with stress when it comes to your weight loss goals, and even your overall health, is when cortisol levels remain consistently high over a long period of time. This is known as chronic stress. This kind of stress is responsible for a whole host of issues including but not limited to:

- decreased bone density
- insulin resistance
- inflammation
- digestive issues
- weight gain
- increased blood pressure
- suppressed immune system

Stress is also detrimental to your sleep. If you're not getting proper, restful sleep, then you risk lowering your ability to burn fat effectively. Your body does most of its repair and recovery when you rest. If your sleep hygiene is not where it needs to be, you can increase your risk of physical injuries, increase cravings for high fat and high sugar foods, decrease your ability to fight of viruses, and decrease your motivation.

***Signs/Symptoms to Look For:***

- You find yourself eating high fat or high sugar foods when stressed
- You find it difficult to unwind at night or get restful sleep

- You constantly feel overwhelmed

- You find it hard for you to recover mentally or physically on your rest days

## 4. Fixed Mindset

A fixed mindset is when you look at a given situation and put a limit on what you believe is possible or can be accomplished. You tend to give more power and credit to the things you can't control instead of focusing on the things you can control.

For example, we know that an individuals genetics only account for about 5% of their results. This means that even if obesity runs in your family, you have more than 95% control over whether or not you end up obese yourself. However, if you've been struggling with overweight or obesity for a long time and then compare yourself to other family members who've been struggling with obesity, a fixed mindset would tell you that there's no way to overcome obesity.

When you have a fixed mindset, you're less likely to push yourself to try new things and more likely to easily give up when something feels hard. You tend to project your past failures into your current reality instead of learning from your past mistakes and recognizing how far you've already come. Under a fixed mindset, you look at your circumstances and make excuses as to why they can't change instead of looking at your circumstances and asking yourself, *"what can be changed?"*.

If you struggle with having a fixed mindset, you need to be very careful with your self-talk. Avoid saying things like:

- "I can *never* seem to..."

- "This *always* happens to me!"

- "*No matter* what I do..."

- "There's *no point* in trying because..."

- "I've *tried everything* and it seems like *nothing* works!"

- "*I can't...*" or "*It's not possible* for me to..."

When you constantly use language that tells yourself what's *not possible* or what you *can't do*, you only reinforce those limitations to become true for you. In the context of weight loss and fitness, when you have a fixed mindset you become less open-minded about exploring new ways to help you achieve your goal. You will have a tendency to shoot down ideas that promote different exercises and nutrition strategies because you believe that the outcome will probably end up in failure.

### *Signs/Symptoms to Look For:*

- You struggle with adopting new tools or strategies because you feel they won't work for you

- You tend to get discouraged and think you're program is failing if you don't see immediate results

- You believe lack of time, genetics, and environment are major factors that hold you back from your weight loss goals

- You feel like your health struggles are due to many things that are out of your control

## 5. Adaptation

Change is hard, yet it's one of the few things that remains constant. If you're trying to lose weight and stay fit for life, you should always be prepared to make lifestyle changes, but more importantly, be patient enough to allow your body the time to adapt to those changes. Most people underestimate how long change can take when it comes to seeing results. If you expect to see lasting results from going on and off some detox, cleanse, diet program, or fitness regimen for a few months at a time and then go back to your old habits, then you will always struggle to see and maintain results.

You've probably heard somewhere that it takes about 21 days to build a new habit, however this is a myth. This was a popular theory back in the 60's and then became really popular leading up to 2015, but truth is that it generally takes more time for a repeated activity or routine to become a habit. Studies show that a habit can form in as little as 18 days or take as long as 254 days, however the average is around 66 days. That means for most people it can take around two months for them to form a new habit—not the typical 21 days.

Even if you manage to form a new healthy habit within three months, you still need to maintain it for at least six months to a year, which is where more than 80% of people begin to relapse back into old, unhealthy habits. Then, if you're fortunate enough to make it through year one, you still need to make it through year five before you can feel confident that your new habits will last a lifetime.

Don't get me wrong, I like the idea of a "21-day" or "30-day" challenges or cleanse, but if you're trying to keep the weight off for good, then you can't stop there. It's like jumping a dead car battery. When your car battery dies, you need to get some juice or another power source to get your car up and running in the right direction. However, if you don't make it a priority to get a new battery then it's only a matter of time before the old battery dies again and you're back at square one.

So, in comparison, I like think of those types of challenges or cleanses as more of a "lifestyle jumpstart". The challenge serves as motivation to get you going in the right direction for the next twenty-one or thirty days. But, if you're not actively working to make permanent lifestyle changes (i.e. change out your old car battery), then you'll always feel stuck and make no progress.

### *Signs/Symptoms to Look For:*

- You tend to participate in programs or challenges that take less than three months to complete

- You find yourself going back to old habits once a program is over

- You find it hard to adopt a new habit for more than six months

- You like programs that require very little changes to your current lifestyle

## 6. Lack of Accountability

When you don't have a strong accountability system in place, you lose one of the strongest predictors of long-term weight loss success.

According to the National Weight Control Registry, people who have lost more than thirty pounds and kept the weight off for more than a year, greatly attribute their results to frequent weight monitoring, ongoing support, and consistent routines. Over a 5-year period, about 5% of people who start a weight loss program will be successful if they attempt it on their own, while about 95% will either quit within a year or regain all of the weight lost within 5 years.

On the other hand, having the right support network, accountability, and boundaries in place, the likelihood of success jumps to 20-35% over five years! Most of the research shows that you are 2-3x more likely to be successful with long-term weight loss if you have the right accountability than someone who tries to do everything on his or her own.

This does not mean that you are not capable of reaching your weight loss or fitness goals on your own. The data just shows that if you lack a strong support system or progress tracking tools, it can be very difficult to maintain your success over a long period of time. Accountability doesn't take away your independence. It helps reinforce the behaviors that make you successful.

***Signs/Symptoms to Look For:***

- You rarely share you health goals with others
- You find it difficult to track your progress on a regular basis
- You find it easy to dismiss certain health-related tasks
- You have a hard time sticking to goals you set for yourself

## 7. Lack of Dietary Alignment

If you are eating primarily for weight loss and not for long-term health, you will never be able to keep your weight where you want it to be. The diet and weight loss industry knows this very well, which is why it's a growing market worth over $90 billion as of 2025.

Millions of people each year participate in various diet programs for the sake of weight loss only for them to fall off and gain it all back in six months. What's heartbreaking is that these same people will repeat this cycle for up to fifteen years without any evidence of long-term success. If you have experienced anything like this yourself, then you would agree that is a very long time for you to waste in order for you to not have control over your weight.

This long and vicious cycle most people experience, also known as "yo-yo dieting", can seriously damage your metabolism, your confidence, your physical health, and even your mental health. When you have a lack of dietary alignment you tend to struggle with poor eating habits, choose poor quality foods, and struggle to figure out what foods are considered "healthy".

One of the best ways I've found to overcome this obstacle is to define the role diet plays in your life. Instead of searching for a diet built around your preferences, you create a more sustainable diet built around your purpose. In other words, if you can figure out how your eating habits will align with your overall health goals currently and in the future, you will discover a way of eating that will naturally lead to long-term weight loss.

### *Signs/Symptoms to Look For:*

- You have tried to lose weight with three or more diet programs within the past five years

- You have a hard time understanding or tracking your macronutrient intake

- You are unsure of how nutrition plays a role in your overall health beyond your weight loss goal

- You feel your diet is generally restrictive and you tend to look forward to cheat meals/days

### **Key Takeaways:**

- 95% of people fail their weight loss attempts within five years because they falsely believe the problem is just lack of motivation or lack or discipline.

- Awareness is the start. Recognize the signs for which obstacles are holding you back and think about what you *could* do to work through those obstacles.

- Remember the **PITFALL**'s: **P**oor Plan, **I**nconsistency, **T**ension, **F**ixed Mindset, **A**daptation, **L**ack of Accountability, **L**ack of Dietary Alignment

Now that you know the obstacles that have been getting in your way, it's time to look at the principles that fit and healthy people live by everyday that not only gets them results, but allows them to keep those results for life.

\*\*\*

For quick access to resources and additional guidance for the material, scan the QR code:

## Chapter Two

# The Principle of Mindset

"For as he thinks in his heart, so is he."

-Proverbs 23:7

"Whether you think you can, or you can't —you're right."

-Henry Ford

Any goal you're working towards, no matter how large or small it seems, will feel impossible to reach with the wrong mindset. When it comes to losing weight and keeping it off, there are some people who can make the right mental shift and see a transformation within months. However, for the majority, this shift can become a struggle that lasts for years, if the shift even happens at all.

So, what is mindset and how do you make the *right* mental shift? Most people believe that in order to have the right mindset you need to have a positive attitude. Although that's definitely an important factor, mindset is more than just positive thoughts and feelings. Mindset is how you interpret your reality. It determines what you believe to be true and influences your behavior in ways that reinforce those beliefs.

For example, if you believe weight loss is hard because you can't seem to stick to a diet for more than ninety days, then you'll behave in a way that sabotages the next diet you try because you'll expect it not to last more than ninety days. Likewise, if you believe that weight loss is hard *but it could be easier* if you found a way to stick to a diet for more than ninety days, then you'll behave in a way that's more solution-seeking than self-sabotaging. How you frame the question in your head can be the difference between success and failure.

## The Power of Perception

In the 1940's, during WWII, many countries including the U.S. experienced shortages with certain medications—particularly morphine, due to Nazi Germany bombing medical supply stations. Morphine, a very powerful painkiller, was often used by soldiers during the war to give them quick pain relief from serious injuries they received during combat. It was also used by doctors as a pre-anesthetic to help calm the patients in preparation for a surgical procedure.

An American anesthesiologist by the name of Dr. Henry Beecher, would frequently be affected by these morphine shortages. This was a problem because he knew that if he were to operate on a soldier without giving them some kind of pain relief, then the overwhelming stress response from the pain could potentially send the soldier into a cardiac shock, where the heart would have a difficult time pumping blood to the rest of the body. This, among other things, could potentially lead to death on the operating table.

As the story goes, Dr. Beecher was preparing to amputate a soldier until he realized that he had run out of morphine. At that moment, he decided to try something a little different. Instead of telling the soldier that they ran out of morphine, he offered the soldier a saline solution (a saltwater mixture) as if it were morphine.

He feared that the soldier would still go into cardiac shock because he knew that the saline solution had no properties to relieve the pain. However, what he had discovered was that the soldier he ended up operating on reported that they felt very little pain! After his initial discovery, Dr Beecher would continue to operate on wounded soldiers and offer a saline solution as an alternative for pain medication whenever morphine supply ran out.

Later in his findings, Dr. Beecher reported that roughly 30-40% of his patients responded favorably to the "fake morphine". That's roughly a third to almost half of the people he operated on reported that they experienced *some* sort of pain relief despite the fact that they actually didn't receive any pain medication!

Basically, what was happening was that when he told his patients that the solution could possibly ease their pain, the patients' mind created a sense of relief in their body that allowed them to behave in a calm manner during the operation. At the time, he was offering what we would call a placebo and his patients were experiencing what is called the "placebo effect".

A placebo is basically a fake drug, treatment, or medication that has no therapeutic or physiological benefit, but has a look or response that's identical to the real thing. The "placebo effect" describes what happens when a person's psychological state produces a physiological response that mimics the positive effects of a drug or treatment as if they had actually received it.

As crazy as this sounds, this phenomenon happens quite often in the field of Medicine. This is just one example that shows how powerful the mind is at producing a positive outcome when you perceive a situation as favorable or you believe something is possible.

But what would happen if you perceive your situation as something negative?

## The Nocebo Effect

In a 2017 study conducted out of Stanford University, researchers performed a histamine skin prick test on the forearm of each participant that produced a mildly irritated rash. They then divided all the participants into two groups where both groups were given a cream to apply onto the rash.

One group was told that the cream was supposed to help improve the rash while the other group was told that the cream might irritate the rash. What they didn't tell the participants was that the cream for both groups actually didn't contain any ingredients that could make the rash better or make it worse.

The purpose of this experiment was to see if the response to a placebo could be manipulated simply by changing the expectations of the participants.

Funny enough, the group that was told that the cream would help with the rash, saw an improvement while the other group that was told that the cream would increase irritation, became irritated and anxious and saw their rash get worse. The effect that works counter to the placebo effect, meaning when your body produces an *unfavorable* physiological response due to *negative* psychological expectations, is called the "nocebo" effect.

By now this shouldn't surprise you, but what made this experiment interesting was that the mind of the participants was literally the only thing that determined what the outcomes would be. There are many other studies and stories that show how your mentality can greatly influence both desired and undesired outcomes, but what lesson are we learning here and what does any of this mean for you?

## Beware of the Fixed Mindset

The principle behind mindset is this: ***behavior follows belief***. Your actions, and ultimately your results, can be directly tied to what you perceive and believe.

To be clear, I'm not talking about "manifestation" or mind over matter. I'm talking about making subtle shifts in the way you view yourself, your health, and your fitness goals because your body will always react and do what it hears your mind say.

Just like in the skin prick test, your belief can be self-sabotaging. I can recall training a licensed therapist back in Boston, who struggled with this. In one of our sessions, she confessed that because she felt she worked really hard in the gym, she deserved to eat whatever she wanted as a reward, which in this case was fast food. For someone who has a deeper understanding of psychology, she understood that her previous way of thinking was sabotaging her results. It was weight loss one week and weight gain the next.

Then there are times where your belief can be self-limiting. At some point, you may have looked back at failed weight loss attempts and assumed that because something didn't work for you in the past then it's likely not going to work for you in the future. Despite there probably being a few successful moments you could've learned from in that previous attempt, you end up throwing the baby out with the bathwater and overlook the wisdom that could help you become successful in your next attempt.

Any belief that says you can't accomplish something because something else is in your way, is what we call a **limiting belief**. Limiting beliefs will make you doubt your fitness program because you'll believe it's too hard. Limiting beliefs will make you feel anxious and stressed when you're three months out from your friend's wedding and you don't think you can lose those extra ten pounds in time. Limiting beliefs increase your lack of motivation, which leads to you skipping workouts, stress eating, and refusing to put forth effort. A pessimist will seldom make progress and doubters often lack determination. As long as your beliefs create doubt about your ability to reach your goals, those beliefs will continue to affect you negatively.

When your belief becomes negative, it can produce negative thoughts, which produce negative feelings, which produce negative behaviors, which produce negative results, which creates negative experiences that reinforce those negative beliefs. This self-sabotaging cycle continues until you decide to make a mental shift that changes it.

This kind of belief usually comes from having a "fixed mindset". A fixed mindset will tell you that obesity or being overweight will always be an issue for you because it runs in the family. A fixed mindset will tell you to avoid lower body workouts because you have "bad knees" or a "bad back". A fixed mindset will tell you to go ahead and eat whatever you want because it's hard to eat the right foods.

And what typically happens when those thoughts creep in? You give up on trying to lose weight; you look for the "easy" exercises to do instead of the ones that actually help you burn calories more effectively; you binge on every sweet thing you can find in your pantry.

## Adopting the Growth Mindset

So, how do we get our mind to work for us and not against us? In short, I believe the answer is to be intentional about looking for the positives and the possibilities in every circumstance. We also need to be careful about how we reframe our past and present experiences. Instead of thinking of failed experiences as something that defines us, we can think of them as moments to learn from and drive us to do better. This is what we call having a **growth mindset**.

A growth mindset will tell you that although obesity runs in the family, your genes only account for about 5% or less of your fitness results. Therefore, you control how much weight you want to lose. A growth mindset will have you think to yourself, "although certain lower body exercises cause my knees to hurt or my back pain to flare up, what alternative exercises or modifications could I make to still target those muscles and achieve the same result?" A growth mindset will recognize that although you messed up on your diet today, it's not the end of the world and you can still bounce back tomorrow.

I would also add that doing a little future planning is important for adopting a growth mindset. Let me ask you this: what does your fit body look like to you besides just losing weight? How long would it realistically take you to reach that goal? Do you have an idea of what your health will look like five years from now?

If you don't have the answers right now, that's okay. We'll figure that out when we get to Chapter 6. For now, you're ahead of the curve because most people haven't even considered any of these questions at all. Most people couldn't even begin to tell you what they wanted their health to look like five weeks from today, much less five years.

Because most people don't consider those questions, it's no coincidence that about 85% of adults will fail to reach their fitness goals within the first year. In addition, less than 10% of those who make it past the first year, will not make it past year five. Which means, out of a hundred people who intend to lose weight, get in shape, and keep their fit lifestyle, about five individuals will make it past year five and get to keep their results for life. Most people don't *plan* for long-term success which is why they don't get long-term results.

## Time to Reframe

If you've been struggling with your mindset up until this point, then I would like for you to make a commitment today to start reframing how you see your negative experiences or past failures. Start asking yourself, "what could I have done differently?" or "what could I do differently now?" If you could see the fit body version of yourself five years from now, what would that version of *you* be doing? If it seems reasonable, then try copying those behaviors today and maybe instead of waiting five years, you can start seeing results in five months!

Keep this in mind: your transformation can accelerate with the right mindset, but can also be ruined with the wrong mindset.

This is why one of the most important things you can do in order to reach your fit body goals, even before you jump into a diet or follow a fitness program, is to choose how you frame your thinking. How do you see your current situation in relation to your goals? What do you believe are the possibilities in relation to your problems? Do you want your fit body to be a fantasy or for real? Are the obstacles you're facing dead ends or detours? However you choose to frame it, I can assure you of this one thing: whatever you believe is true, your behavior will follow through.

### Key Takeaways:

- Behavior follows belief—You will usually behave and do whatever it is you perceive to be true.

- Negative beliefs produce negative thoughts, which leads to negative actions and behaviors.

- A fixed mindset is self-sabotaging while a growth mindset is solution-seeking.

- A fixed mindset makes you focus on things you can't control by emphasizing your past negative experiences and/or failures. A growth mindset makes you focus on the things you *can* control and emphasizes opportunities for you to learn and try things different from your previous experiences.

Although mindset can be a very powerful catalyst for change, what do you do when it seems like you're doing all the right things but your body *still* doesn't want to cooperate? In the next chapter, we'll look at a principle that stresses the importance of creating healthy habits and why creating the *right* environment is just as, if not more, important as the habits themselves.

***

For quick access to resources and additional guidance for the material, scan the QR code:

# Chapter Three
# The Principle of Function

"A person is either the effect of his environment or is able to have an effect upon his environment."
-L. Ron Hubbard

Does your lifestyle allow for weight loss to feel *natural* or do you feel like you need to *force* it to happen? In other words, is weight loss the byproduct of your lifestyle or is it the main focus?

## The "Biggest Loser" Study

In 2016, a paper was published in the journal *Obesity* that followed up with fourteen individuals six years after they had competed on the hit reality TV weight loss show called *The Biggest Loser*. The premise of the show was to take individuals who were obese and, within a 30-week timeframe, get them to lose as much weight as possible.

The show accomplished this by putting contestants through a severe caloric deficit (around a 1,200-calorie diet) and then had them do high intensity training for ninety minutes a day, six days a week. To give you some reference, the safe upper limit for weight loss for the average person would be about two pounds per week. This means that within thirty weeks, the average person should lose anywhere between 30 to 60 pounds. However, in the show, contestants saw an average weight loss of about 128 pounds! That averages to weight loss of about 4.3 pounds per week—more than double the upper limit of what we would consider safe weight loss.

## Short-term Reward, Long-term Ruin

Given the nature of the show, researchers wanted to know how well these participants maintained their weight loss in the real world, more than five years after their season was over. What they found was that all but one of the contestants had regained around 70% or more of the weight they lost, which translated to about 90 pounds of weight regain.

Overall, you could say that the contestants maintained *some* weight loss, however they weren't able to do it well. In fact, mostly every contestant suffered long-term metabolic damage because of the way they approached weight loss on the show. Here are just three majors factors that were negatively impacted:

1) ***Metabolism*** - Contestants had their resting metabolic rate (i.e: the rate at which your body burns calories at rest) drop significantly. They were burning on average 500 to 800 *less* calories each day than what they used to burn when they were heavier. This meant that their bodies were actively fighting against further weight loss.

2) ***Muscle Loss*** - Lean muscle is very important when it comes to your metabolism and burning calories, especially when you're at rest. On the show, the high intensity training the contestants participated in was more cardio-based than weight lifting. Due to the excessive cardio, their bodies were breaking down muscle tissue as well as fat for energy. As a consequence, they hurt their body's metabolism and lowered their ability to burn more calories at rest.

3) ***Hormonal Disruption*** - Leptin is a hormone that tells your brain that your body is full. Before the show, all the contestants had fairly normal leptin levels, however during the follow-up, researchers discovered that the contestants had very low leptin levels. This meant that they experienced stronger signals for hunger and decreased food satisfaction, which made them want to consume more calories than they normally would.

After many client conversations and consultations, I've discovered that most people don't want to lose weight too fast because they sort of understand how unhealthy that can be. However, despite what some of them tell me, they *still* approach weight loss in the exact same manner as those who competed on this show–just not as extreme.

Most people go on a low calorie diet, workout hard by doing more cardio, and then go back to their old lifestyles expecting to keep their new results. Weight loss done this way just isn't sustainable and your body will almost always fight against it.

## Form Follows Function

So, how do you get your body to stop fighting against you and start working with you? I believe it starts with understanding this principle: **your form will follow your functions**. To put it another way, your body will generally reflect or adapt to your current lifestyle and the environments that you regularly associate with.

If you change the way things function in your environment, your lifestyle and your body will adapt to that change. For example, if your current environment promotes a sedentary lifestyle and you spend eight hours a day seated at a desk, then your body will reflect that through increased fat stores in the midsection, tight hips, poor posture, and a weak back. If you want your body to change, then you need to put yourself in an environment where you're encouraged to strengthen your body, your posture, and burn more calories.

A healthy body requires healthy habits. Healthy habits require a healthy environment. Another example is junk food snacking. If you want to stop eating junk food then don't bring any junk food into your home environment. In health coaching, we call this **stimulus control**. This is when you either add or remove certain things in your environment in order to trigger a certain behavior.

With that being said, here's what I don't want you to miss: when you're trying to adopt healthy habits that promote weight loss, it is extremely important that you try to make those habits *feel natural* and easy to do. If the change is too drastic or feels too overwhelming, then your body is going to fight hard to reject it.

After all, that was one of the issues with most of the contestants from *The Biggest Loser*. Yes, the environment on the show *did* enable them to lose weight and be more active instead of sedentary, however that lifestyle didn't feel natural for them in the real world. As a result, mostly everyone was unable to keep up with the high-intensity activities and low-calorie diet that got them success in the first place.

## The One That "Got It Right"

Before I close this chapter, I do want to talk about the *one* contestant in that study that actually did well in maintaining their weight loss long-term and how you can use their success to your advantage:

1) ***Healthy Weight Range*** - As mentioned before, due to the way that the show approached weight loss, a small amount of weight did come back but not much. Instead of trying to hold onto the unrealistic weight loss they initially reached on the show, the individual found a healthy weight range that they could safely maintain with the lifestyle they wanted. They shifted their focus from having weight loss be the goal, to being the byproduct of maintaining a healthy lifestyle.

2) ***New Body, New Standards*** - While most contestants tried to take their new bodies into their old lifestyle, this contestant decided to change their lifestyle to keep their new body. This individual created systems in their life that kept their hunger and metabolism in check in order to prevent weight gain from getting out of control.

3) ***Sustainable Habits*** - In order to keep the new standard, the contestant adopted certain weight loss habits they picked up from the show and found ways to make it more practical with their lifestyle such as meal planning, calorie and behavior tracking, scheduled fitness activities, and so on. These habits gave the contestant a better sense of control over their health outcomes, which also increased lifestyle satisfaction and overall well-being.

4) ***Increased Activity*** - This individual still did moderate to intense physical activity for more than an hour each day, which was close to what they used to do when they were on the show. This allowed them to continue to burn calories at rest despite the fact that their metabolism slowed down like everyone else's.

The main point here is that in order to keep the results, some permanent changes need to be made in order to meet the demands of your new body. The process is not going to feel comfortable at first, but if you give it some time, your body will adjust to the "new" normal.

In summary, it's not sustainable to think that you can lose weight fast over a short period of time and to keep it off over a long period of time. Not only do you experience burnout quicker doing it this way, but you can cause long-term damage to your body both physically and metabolically. Instead, set the lifestyle you want as the standard and then let your physical, mental, and social environments meet that new standard. Remember: when the environment changes, the body adapts. Form follows function.

> **Key Takeaways:**
>
> - Your lifestyle is a direct reflection of the environment you create. **Form follows function**. Change the way things function in your life and you'll change your lifestyle to reach your fitness goals.
>
> - Take a close look at your physical, mental, and social influences and analyze how they either positively or negatively impact your weight loss.
>
> - Make manageable and sensible changes; don't try to do too much too fast or your body will fight against it.
>
> - It sounds counterintuitive but if weight loss is your focus, it'll be hard to maintain long-term; if lifestyle is your focus, weight loss will be *easier* to maintain long-term.

Creating an environment that promotes healthy weight loss is great, but what good is it if you let your eating habits undo all of your progress? That's why in this next chapter, we're going to look at a principle that will help you avoid the common mistakes found in most diets and show you which kinds of foods naturally promote long-term weight loss.

\*\*\*

For quick access to resources and additional guidance for the material, scan the QR code:

## Chapter Four
# The Principle of Diet

"Your diet is your bank account. Good food choices are good investments.

-Bethenny Frankel

You can't outwork a poor diet. I've had clients in the past who have tried almost everything to lose weight: CrossFit$^{TM}$, P90X$^{TM}$, appetite suppressants, fat burners, and even surgery. Sooner or later, when the weight eventually comes back, they realize what you eat is just as important, if not more important, than what you do.

Generally speaking, nutrition accounts for about 70-80% of your results. If you get everything else right but keep making poor dietary choices, then long-term weight loss will feel like a goal you can never accomplish. You'll always be stuck in this cycle of frustration where you feel like you're constantly taking one step forward and five steps backward.

Diet is one of the most important factors to your fitness, weight loss, and overall health, you can not afford to overlook. So, what *should* you eat? What foods or eating habits are sabotaging your efforts? Can you find the "right" diet to stick with or are you just setting yourself up for a lifetime of disappointment?

## The Truth About Weight Gain From The World's Most Dangerous Restaurant

Would you believe me if I told you that there is a restaurant in the U.S. where the menu and the food are intentionally designed to damage your body and clog your arteries? It's probably not at all that unbelievable. However, at this particular establishment they take it a couple steps further. They have a sign at the front door telling you that the food here *is* bad for your health.

If you decided that you were going to ignore that sign and become a patron at your own risk, you would put on a hospital gown, check in on the scale, and order menu items with names like "Quadruple Bypass" and "Triple Bypass Burger". With your burger, you could order an endless side of "Flatliner Fries" that are deep fried in pure lard and covered in chili and cheese. For dessert, you can get full-fat ice cream and a milkshake loaded with heavy cream.

You would not be able to order anything considered "healthy" such as a side salad or even a leaf of lettuce for your burger. You also would not be able to find anything on the menu that is low-calorie because virtually everything they offer is extremely high in fat.

This may sound like a glutton's paradise, but what if the owner of this particular restaurant came up to you and said, "If you eat the food here, you will die." – then points to a table where he has the cremated remains of a customer who died of a heart attack moments after eating his food? Would you listen to him or awkwardly laugh him off? Now, would you believe me if I told you that the owner of this establishment, that has been dubbed, "The World's Most Dangerous Restaurant", at one point used to be a fitness coach who owned and operated a chain of health clubs?

His name is Jon Basso, and after spending many years in the fitness industry helping people lose weight, he slowly began feeling like it was all pointless. He felt like he couldn't be honest in his approach to delivering weight loss results for his clients because no matter what he tried, he could not stop them from cheating on their diets and ruining their progress. As he was going through this internal struggle, Jon ended up in a huge legal battle with a well-known restaurant where he was forced to shut down his health clubs and nearly lost everything.

Instead of giving up, he took whatever little money he had left, and decided he was going to create his own restaurant. His goal wasn't just to get back at the same entity that almost took him down, but he wanted to build a brand that he felt was going to represent being brutally honest to himself and his customers.

Jon decided he was going to lean into the frustrations he was experiencing with his former clients around their food choices of and wanted his restaurant to prove a point: that people *will* overeat and gain weight when they are exposed to foods that are designed to maximize fat and calorie intake. He even went as far as to call out other restaurants on national television by saying that they don't have the integrity to warn customers to their faces and tell them that the food they serve is just as unhealthy as his. In addition, he also tells his customers that eating this kind of food long enough will lead to very serious, or even fatal consequences.

And with that honesty, his single restaurant has been estimated to bring in more money each year than three Burger King's combined. He didn't open this restaurant to accidentally serve high-calorie food, he purposely wanted to exploit the body's biology through food without hiding it from you. And the cremated remains he keeps in his restaurant? It's the tragic proof that he isn't lying about his product. It serves as a reminder that his customers keep giving him informed consent and that they will continue to risk their lives at the expense of the food they enjoy; the same food he keeps warning them not to eat. Now, I know this sounds like some twisted, personal trainer supervillain origin story, and I wish this was all made up, but sadly it's true.

What's interesting is that if some people appreciate his honesty enough to still eat at his establishment knowing the risks, then you'd figure more people would appreciate the advice he gave in a 2012 interview where he says, "...if you just get good sleep, avoid alcohol, and eat fruits and vegetables, you will be as healthy as you can be".

## Food Isn't Neutral

I definitely do not condone nor respect the ethics behind this man's business. However, as perverted as his philosophy and methods may seem, the one thing I can respect about him is his honesty. When it comes to the topic of food and dieting, we tend to disregard the truth that's right in front of us in order to justify our preferences.

His story illustrates an obvious but frequently debated truth: *food is not neutral.* Some foods move your body toward better health, balance, and leanness while others can push you toward overeating, fat gain, metabolic imbalance, and long-term health complications.

This chapter isn't about creating a meal plan or telling you *exactly* what foods you need to eat. It's about understanding the *principle* at play because once you see how food affects your body, making consistently healthy choices becomes far easier.

## The Diet Deception

When it comes to dieting, here's the uncomfortable truth: diets both succeed and fail. To be clear, I'm talking about the popular diets that are promoted primarily for weight loss. These diets succeed because, more often than not, they give you the weight loss you're looking for. Practically every diet is designed to shock your system in the beginning phases with calorie reduction and water loss, which allows you to see weight changes quickly, feel good, and make you believe that you've "fixed" the diet problem.

But after that phase goes away, weight loss seems to plateau and you stop seeing results. This is where diets fail because almost all of them are designed for short-term relief and not long-term transformation. Once the diet ends, old habits (and often old foods) return. The weight comes back, sometimes more than before, and the body rebounds, just like from *The Biggest Loser*. Over a 6-month period, diets on average have a less than 20% success rate. If you look at a 5-year period, diets have a 5% success rate and over a 10-year period, that number drops to 1%.

By accepting that many diets are selling relief, and not lasting change, you can break free from this trap of losing weight and gaining it all back. The real work starts not in restriction, but in understanding and building sustainable habits that are opposite of what most people are doing. Now, let's look at some myths you may have been exposed to that are having you fall for the diet deceptions.

## The 4 Diet Myths

Here are what I consider the four most common myths (or at least half-truths) that I think keep people confused and stuck in this seemingly endless dieting cycle:

## Myth #1: All calories are created equal.

On paper, a calorie is just a unit of energy, but in the human body, not all calories behave equally. Why? Because foods differ dramatically in: fiber content, water content, processing, how quickly they digest, how they affect hunger and satiety hormones, and how satisfying they are. For example, 100 calories from oil or butter will generally leave you hungry soon after you consume it while 100 calories from a high-fiber vegetable or legume will stretch your stomach, trigger fullness signals, and sustain you longer.

In studies that link actual eating behavior to weight gain, these differences matter a lot. When you treat all calories the same, you miss the bigger picture and make the mistake of justifying junk food bingeing on your cheats days because you're only focused on the calorie number and not the content of where the calories come from. The quality and food structure of calories matters.

## Myth #2: Low-carb diets cause fat loss because carbs make you fat.

This is one of the most pervasive diet myths that I wish would die. Sadly, because it has a grain (or two) of truth, the lie is even more seductive. More accurately, highly processed carbs, especially in excess, can make you fat. When you compound those kinds of carbs with dietary fat, then being overweight or obese is almost a sure result.

You will often see rapid weight loss when you go low-carb, which can create the assumption that carbs were "the problem" however, much of the early weight loss on a low-carb diet comes from water, it's not from fat. When carbohydrate intake drops, your body burns through stored glycogen (the storage form of glucose in the muscle and liver). Each gram of glycogen holds several grams of water. Once glycogen is used, the water quickly disappears. In short, you lose "water weight."

Additionally, carb restriction is often paired with reduced overall food intake (due to reduced appetite or food options), which can lower calories. So, the fat loss is largely from reduced total energy intake, not because carbs were the enemy all along.

What's truly sad about this myth is that most dieters, and even some of my clients, will often avoid fruits and some vegetables because of the "carbs" even though there's not a *single* study to prove that fruits and vegetables, *even consumed in excess*, are associated with weight gain. In fact, every single study you find on vegetables, and especially fruits, is positively associated with weight loss![1] But alas, because certain media channels promote misinformation about carbs, fear and lies get to run around the world before the truth can put on its shoes.

## Myth #3: You can eat high-fat foods to burn fat.

High-fat, low-carb diets have been around for a long time, however the recent resurgence of the Ketogenic Diet has since popularized this idea that by eating more fat, you burn more fat as fuel. But while fat is efficient for energy, it is the most calorie-dense macronutrient at 9 calories per gram versus 4 calories per gram for both carbs and protein.

That density means you can consume a lot of energy with very little volume. When you eat high-fat foods, especially processed fats, oils, cheese, and fried foods, it's easy to overconsume fat calories without realizing it, thus making it incredibly easy to put on weight. The restaurant owner's story mentioned before openly exploits this fact when he created his menu.

To prove to my clients that their weight loss struggle may be a result of overconsumption of fat, I give them a small assignment (this assignment is also outlined in Chapter 8) to track their calories for a week in order to see where their total calories come from. Almost all of them find that they overconsume fat and underconsume carbs without realizing. High-fat eating is pretty "efficient" if you're trying to store or maintain weight, not lose it.[2]

## Myth #4: Protein is the most important nutrient for weight loss.

Almost every fitness enthusiast or expert will say this about protein: 1) if you want to gain weight and muscle, eat more protein. 2) If you want to lose weight and save muscle, eat more protein. And although the advice is not technically wrong, it can lead to a way of eating that will become problematic later.

In many people's eyes, protein is king. When you mention protein, people naturally think of animal protein as the only "real" source of protein and every other form of protein is "incomplete" or inferior. The issue with this kind of thinking is that most animal protein sources that people consume (such as red meat, pork, sausage, full-fat dairy products, etc.) are high in fat, especially saturated fat, which is associated with weight gain. Therefore, if eating more protein is your focus but you neglect eating lean, you can certainly overconsume the fat calories that come with that kind of protein.

Protein has legitimate benefits: satiety (feeling of fullness), muscle preservation, thermic effect (the amount of energy your body uses during digestion), and metabolic maintenance. But diets that overemphasize protein and neglect fiber, water, and volume, often still fail because fat loss and healthy body composition come from overall proper dietary habits, not protein alone.

If you eat high-protein but low-fiber, high-fat, highly processed meals, you may preserve muscle but body fat can still accumulate. In short, protein is an important nutrient for weight loss, but it's not everything and you certainly don't need as much of it as you think you do unless you're a competitive athlete.

## The Culprits Behind Weight Struggle

Now that we've looked at some of the myths, I want to address the two biggest culprits I believe play a big role in the struggle with weight loss, especially if you are consuming a more modern, western diet. There are other factors and situations to consider when it comes to why some people struggle with their diet to lose weight, but we're focusing on these two because we live in a society where access and consumption of these foods are very high.

## Culprit #1: Ultra-Processed Foods (UPFs)

This may seem like an obvious one, but when I say ultra-processed foods (UPF) I'm referring to packaged snacks, sweet or savory processed items, frozen meals, sugary cereals, processed meats, many fast-food items, and basically most of the highly accessible foods that are engineered for addictive taste, convenience, and long shelf-life.

There is strong evidence that supports the link between high UPF consumption and weight gain or obesity. For example, in a 2021 study, nearly 350,000 people across nine countries in Europe found that those who consumed the highest amounts of UPF's had a 15% greater risk of becoming overweight over five years.[3] In another study, researchers found that participants who consumed UPF's consumed about 500 more calories per day than participants who consumed foods that were minimally processed. Within a two-week period, the participants who consumed UPF's, gained roughly 2 pounds whereas the other group lost about that same amount of weight.[4]

These kinds of foods can be found in abundance in the Western Diet (i.e. Standard American Diet) and they are designed to be both highly palatable and calorically dense. These foods often lack nutrients such as fiber and water and are instead packed with alarming amounts of additives, flavorings, fat, sugar, salt, and other chemicals in order to trick your brain into consuming lots of those calories without feeling full.[5]

## Culprit #2: High-Fat Foods and Dairy

We touched on high-fat foods not too long ago and how easy it is to overconsume calories from fat, but something you should also consider is the concentration of calories from fat that comes from dairy, more specifically cheese. In the U.S., cheese is the single largest source of saturated fat intake.

Saturated fats (i.e: fat that can be found in the skin of animal products, fatty red meat, full-fat dairy, lard, and tallow) are considered one of the unhealthy fats (trans fat being the other unhealthy fat) because they typically raise your LDL ("bad cholesterol"), can damage your blood vessels, and can increase your risk of heart disease or stroke. And if that wasn't bad enough, there are some studies that show that high amounts of dietary saturated fat intake is associated with weight gain and higher rates of obesity.[6,7]

The average American now consumes about 41 pounds of cheese per year. To put that in perspective, that would mean that the average American consumes about 5,517g of fat in an entire year from cheese alone. In calories, that would equate to roughly 49,653 calories from fat in a year. Since one pound of fat is roughly 3,500 calories, then theoretically speaking, you could experience up to 14 pounds of fat loss in a year (49,653 kcal/3,500 kcal = 14.18) by simply cutting out cheese.

Once again, I'm just giving you something to consider; this isn't an instruction to start dropping foods from your diet. But, keep in mind the lesson we learned earlier from Jon and his restaurant: he understood the mechanisms behind weight gain and he created his menu intentionally to include excessive amounts of full-fat dairy products and cheese for a reason.

## The Five Components to Diet Success

Hopefully by now, you have an idea of what foods or eating habits are sabotaging your efforts but still, what *should* you eat? What is considered the "best" diet for weight loss and is it sustainable?

Every diet that works long-term, whether it's Mediterranean, Flexitarian, plant-based, low-fat, even some versions of higher-protein diets, they all share *one unifying principle:* **foods that are highly associated with promoting longevity *naturally* lead to a leaner body**. No matter what label the diet uses, the effective versions all have the same characteristics that make up these foods:

**1. Higher fiber** - Fiber regulates appetite, stabilizes blood sugar, and slows digestion. Studies show that volume, fiber, and food structure keep you feeling full for longer periods of time.[8]

**2. Higher water content** - Water-rich foods (vegetables, fruits, legumes, grains) naturally reduce calorie density, contribute to partial hydration, and add volume.[9]

**3. Lower calorie density** - You can eat more food for fewer calories.

**4. Less processing** - Foods closer to their natural state retain more of their micronutrients (such as vitamins, minerals, fiber, antioxidants, phytonutrients, etc.) that help regulate appetite and allow your body to have the proper hormonal responses.

**5. Less added fat** - Especially from highly processed oils, cheese, and fried foods.

This universal principle is why the longest-living populations on Earth, such as those found in the "Blue Zones", naturally maintain lower body weight without having to "diet" in the traditional sense. These populations, who are well-known to have groups of people that live well over 90 years or even 100 years old, eat according to these patterns without having to focus on weight loss partly because they're exposed to foods that make it very difficult to put on excess body fat.

Eating the right foods for sustainable weight loss doesn't have to be complicated. But if you are ignorant about the function of food, then you'll always be a slave to the diet deceptions.

My answer to you is don't worry about trying to find the "best" diet for weight loss, because almost every single diet out there can do that. Instead, look for the best foods and eating patterns that support longevity and you will *by default* find foods associated with weight loss. Longevity equals lean is the equation.

> **Key Takeaways:**
>
> - You can not outwork a bad diet. Poor food choices will eventually catch up to your body.
>
> - Food isn't neutral. What you eat — how processed it is, how calorie-dense, how fiber-rich/water-rich — affects your physiology, hormones, metabolism, appetite, and long-term health.
>
> - Ultra-processed foods (UPF's) and high-fat, calorie-dense foods can be the main culprits behind your struggle with weight loss. Consider limiting or avoiding these kinds of foods.
>
> - Practically every eating pattern that's successful and associated with weight loss and good health, contains foods that offer volume, satiation, low calorie density, and very minimal processing.
>
> - Remember: longevity equals lean

Now that you understand the principle of diet and how certain food can influence your weight and your body, the next step is learning how to build the habits that support lasting change. That's where we're going next.

\*\*\*

For quick access to resources and additional guidance for the material, scan the QR code:

# References

1. Arnotti, Karla, and Mandy Bamber. "Fruit and Vegetable Consumption in Overweight or Obese Individuals: A Meta-Analysis." *Western journal of nursing research* vol. 42,4 (2020): 306-314. doi:10.1177/0193945919858699

2. Warwick, Z S, and S S Schiffman. "Role of dietary fat in calorie intake and weight gain." *Neuroscience and biobehavioral reviews* vol. 16,4 (1992): 585-96. doi:10.1016/s0149-7634(05)80198-8

3. Srour, Bernard, et al. "Ultra-Processed Food Intake and Risk of Overweight and Obesity: The NutriNet-Santé Prospective Cohort Study." *American Journal of Clinical Nutrition*, vol. 114, no. 2, 2021, pp. 441–451

4. Hall, Kevin D., et al. "Ultra-Processed Diets Cause Excess Calorie Intake and Weight Gain: An Inpatient Randomized Controlled Trial of Ad Libitum Food Intake." *Cell Metabolism*, vol. 30, no. 1, 2019, pp. 67–77

5. Rolls, Barbara J. "Dietary Energy Density: Applying Behavioural Science to Weight Management." *Nutrition Bulletin*, vol. 42, no. 3, 2017, pp. 246–253

6. Hariri, Niloofar et al. "A highly saturated fat-rich diet is more obesogenic than diets with lower saturated fat content." *Nutrition research (New York, N.Y.)* vol. 30,9 (2010): 632-43. doi:10.1016/j.nutres.2010.09.003

7. Geng, Tingting et al. "Effects of Dairy Products Consumption on Body Weight and Body Composition Among Adults: An Updated Meta-Analysis of 37 Randomized Control Trials." *Molecular nutrition & food research* vol. 62,1 (2018): 10.1002/mnfr.201700410. doi:10.1002/mnfr.201700410

8. Porrini, M et al. "Effects of physical and chemical characteristics of food on specific and general satiety." *Physiology & behavior* vol. 57,3 (1995): 461-8. doi:10.1016/0031-9384(94)00242-w

9. Rolls, B J. "Dietary energy density: Applying behavioural science to weight management." *Nutrition bulletin* vol. 42,3 (2017): 246-253. doi:10.1111/nbu.12280

# Chapter Five
# The Principle of Discipline

"Discipline is the bridge between goals and accomplishment."

-Jim Rohn

Your next fit body breakthrough will come when you stop relying on motivation and start building momentum to reach your goal through simple, consistent actions that build discipline.

When you apply the first principle of mindset to the principle of discipline, which we'll soon discuss, then your desire to form healthy habits becomes amplified. But first, you need to stop telling yourself that you're not "disciplined" enough.

## The Invisible Muscle

If your body is the vehicle, your mindset is the GPS, and your diet is the fuel, then discipline is the engine. It's the invisible force that turns your intention into reality. It's the deciding factor between the person who *wants* to lose weight and get fit and the person who *decides* to lose weight and become fit. But discipline can be misunderstood.

Most people think discipline is about being tough, being strict, or punishing themselves when they mess up. They imagine Olympic-level self-control, 4 a.m. workouts, and a constant feeling of peak motivation. But that's not discipline…that's a movie version of discipline. In real life, discipline isn't that glamorous. It's more practical and strategic. It's something you have to train, not something you just *have*.

## Discipline Doesn't Remove Difficulty

"Once I'm disciplined, everything will feel easy." is one of the lies most people believe about discipline. Discipline doesn't remove difficulty. It makes you capable of moving through difficult moments. Discipline is more like a capacity, not a comfort zone. Michael Jordan, one of the greatest basketball players ever, didn't practice relentlessly because it was easy. Arnold Schwarzenegger didn't dominate the gym because it felt effortless. Serena Williams didn't become one of the greatest athletes alive because showing up to training was comfortable.

They were all disciplined because they trained the ability to show up, especially when it felt hard.

Discipline is not the absence of struggle. Discipline is the ability to move forward through struggle. Adopting healthy habits is hard, but just because you struggle with them doesn't mean you're failing. In reality, it means that you still may be in the beginning stage of the learning process or what psychologists call the **Hierarchy of Competence**.

## The Hierarchy of Competence

Every skill or habit you've ever learned has gone through four stages:

1. **Unconscious Incompetence** — you don't know what you're bad at

2. **Conscious Incompetence** — you now know what you're bad at and realize it's hard (this is the painful stage)

3. **Conscious Competence** — you know how to do it, but it takes some conscious effort

4. **Unconscious Competence** — you know how to do it almost effortlessly or automatically

If you're like most people, you probably get caught up and quit in stage two. This is the moment when your routines feel unnatural; your workouts feel intimidating; your nutrition feels overwhelming; your progress feels too slow. This stage is where self-doubt creeps in. This is the stage where you really begin to question if what you're doing is worth all the trouble. But here's what elite athletes and the greats understood: discipline is the bridge between stage two (conscious incompetence) and stage four (unconscious competence).

Arnold didn't walk into the gym at 15 years old with amazing technique or perfect form. Michael Jordan didn't jump right onto the varsity team his first year of high school...he was cut. Serena Williams didn't start her career in tennis as the incredible athlete we know today...she trained for a decade before she reached the top of her game.

They all started in stage one. They all struggled through stage two. They all built discipline during stage three. They all eventually reached stage four, which is what we call mastery, but it was the discipline that got them there. And the same thing happens in health and fitness. Every habit begins as something that feels out of place, inconvenient, or difficult.

Discipline is what carries you through that part where it still feels unnatural. The goal is to be able to get you to the point where you can feel confident performing certain exercises in the gym, with good form, and not feel like you'll end up as the next "#gymfail" meme on social media. So, if you feel like you're in the middle of stage two or stage three, rest assured that you're not doing it wrong. You're on the right track. The main principle when it comes to understanding discipline is that: **discipline eases difficulty.**

## Why Consistency Feels Hard

The next thing most people often beat themselves up for is not being "consistent". Consistency usually breaks down if there is too much friction or things in your way that cause you to lose momentum towards your fitness goals. There are four main reasons consistency feels difficult:

### 1. Your habits are untrained

A trained habit is automatic. An untrained habit requires energy, attention, and focus. A trained habit feels easy. An untrained habit feels like a constant struggle.

This is why waking up at the same time every day becomes easier after a month, but feels almost impossible during the first week. This is why eating a nutritious breakfast becomes easy after you've done it for a few weeks, but feels like a chore when you're used to skipping it. If the habit isn't trained yet, consistency will always feel like a fight.

### 2. The habit has too many moving parts

Complexity will kill your consistency. You're setting yourself up for disappointment when you attempt habits that require too much preparation, too much decision-making, too much emotional effort, or too much time. Discipline thrives on clarity and simplicity. Michael Jordan didn't practice "everything" every day. He focused on different areas of his game on different occasions. Arnold's training wasn't random; he knew exactly what body parts he was going to work on each day. Serena Williams didn't improvise her training; she practiced the fundamentals everyday. The simpler your habit, the easier it is to build discipline.

## 3. You don't have enough accountability

Accountability is behavioral reinforcement. It doesn't mean someone is trying to dictate your every move or is "telling you what to do." It means someone or something is helping you stay aligned with what you already want. Accountability helps with follow-through, long-term consistency, motivation, and resilience.

In fact, neuroscience shows that social accountability increases the reward response in the brain, which means you're literally more likely to succeed when someone is supporting you. And as we'll talk about later, accountability is one of the major ingredients in the discipline formula.

## 4. The habit doesn't feel controllable

If a workout routine feels impossible → you'll quit.

If a diet feels restrictive → you'll cheat.

If your schedule feels unpredictable → you'll slack.

This is, in my opinion, the most underrated factor when it comes to discipline. If a task feels out of your control, it will feel impossible for you to stay consistent. People stay consistent with the things they feel *capable* of doing. In short, if you feel that you can't control the behavior, you won't continue the behavior.

## The Discipline Formula

So, how do you get to the point where you can properly build discipline and not feel like you're running into a dead end every time your fitness journey starts to feel hard? If I had to compress the entire concept of discipline into a formula, this would be it:

**Accountability + Persistence + Consistency = Discipline**

## Accountability

Accountability is what provides structure, encouragement, and course correction. It's the external factor that keeps you on track when your internal motivation fails. Remember, it's not someone telling you what to do. Accountability is simply someone or something that's there to give you that extra support and prevent you from falling off track. This could come in the form of:

- a coach
- a doctor
- a friend or family member
- a workout partner
- an app
- a fitness community

It's hard to imagine Michael without Phil Jackson or Arnold without Joe Weider or Serena without King Richard. If the greatest athletes and actors you know have accountability to help them succeed, then the same can and will work for you.

## Persistence

Persistence is the ability to continue even when your progress stops or feels slow, when your motivations drops, when life gets in the way, or when stress increases at work and at home. Persistence is about *keeping momentum*. This is why the best athletes are not the ones who never fail. The best athletes are the ones who fail often. They are the ones who refuse to quit. Arnold lost some keys competitions before he ever won Mr. Olympia. Jordan missed thousands of shots before he became a legend and led the Bulls to win 6, near-consecutive, championships. Serena lost many matches, and struggled with injuries, before winning her 7 singles titles.

When you're persistent, you understand that the number on scale is going to go up a few times before it goes down. You'll run into moments where you'll feel weak during your workouts even if you've done the weights before without any issue. When those moments happen, the response isn't to beat yourself up when failure or obstacles occur. Aim to press forward and see it as an opportunity to win the next day.

## Consistency

Consistency is not about being perfect. It's about showing up regularly and having routines you can rely on. It's about building competence and confidence through repeatable actions every single day. It's about predictability. In order for you to show up, remember that there needs to be low friction and control within your environment.

When you combine accountability, persistence, and consistency, you create the conditions for discipline to improve.

## Time to Dominate Your Health Habits

By now, I hope you can begin to see discipline in a different light and, if this applies to you, maybe you can stop being too hard on yourself about "not having enough discipline". Discipline is the accumulation of trained habits, supported by accountability, executed with persistence, and sustained through consistency. You don't have to wait for motivation to be present in order for you to go after you fitness goals. Focus on creating the conditions that will allow discipline to thrive and, before you know it, those healthy habits will become second nature.

**Key Chapter Takeaways:**

- Discipline isn't something you *have*, it's something you train.

- It took time for all successful athletes and individuals to become disciplined. The same is true when it comes to your health and fitness as well.

- Discipline requires consistency (i.e: doing the same action everyday) plus persistence (i.e: doing the same actions despite difficulties, discouragement, or failure), and accountability (i.e: structure, community, coaching, etc) to keep you on track.

- Consistency feels hard when your habits are untrained, when there are too many moving parts, when there's no accountability, and when you don't feel like you have control.

- Discipline doesn't remove difficulty, it gives you the ability navigate through it. Remember: Discipline eases difficulty.

Now it's time to put these principles into action! In Part II, we're going to tie everything together step-by-step using the F.A.S.T

Method framework. Remember the four principles we discussed in this section:

1. **Behavior follows belief** — Whatever you believe is true, your behavior will follow through.

2. **Form follows function** — Your body will adapt to your lifestyle and environment.

3. **Longevity is lean** — Foods that promote longevity tend to also promote leanness.

4. **Discipline eases difficulty** — The longer you work on your health habits, the easier those habits become.

***

For quick access to resources and additional guidance for the material, scan the QR code:

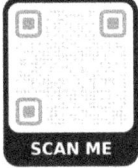

# PART II:
# THE F.A.S.T METHOD

"Plans are successful only to the extent that they can be executed."

-John C. Maxwell


"A good plan is like a road map: it shows the final destination and usually the best way to get there."

-H. Stanley Judd

## Chapter Six

# Focus

"Energy flows where the focus goes."

-Tony Robbins

"The mind always fails first, not the body. The secret is to make the mind work for you, not against you."

-Arnold Schwarzenegger

Up until this point, we've looked at a four key principles that separate those who succeed at reaching their health and fitness goals from those who don't. In Chapter 2, we specifically talked about the importance of having the right mindset and how having this kind of mindset can help you see opportunities to grow and push forward where you would normally see obstacles that would hold you back. In this chapter, you're going to learn how to begin to take those principles and make them practical.

The first step in shaping your fit body and avoiding the weight loss traps that have been keeping you stuck is to sharpen your focus. Much like using a GPS, you need to give your brain a specific place to go in order for it to consciously and subconsciously look for the best path to get there. Sharpening your focus starts by clearly defining your fitness goal.

## Don't Be Like Alice

In the classic story of *Alice in Wonderland,* there's a point in the story where Alice is lost in the woods and she comes across the Cheshire Cat. She asks the cat how to get out of the woods to which the cat replies,"which way would you like to go?". Alice replies by saying that she doesn't care which way just as long as it leads to the way out. The cat then tells Alice that it doesn't matter which way she goes, which leaves her stuck in the same spot.

This answer clearly frustrates Alice because it's not the answer she was looking for, but the point is that she never asked for a *specific* destination and therefore didn't get a specific path to follow.

## The Real Purpose of a Goal

The problem that most people face, like Alice, is that they treat their goals like wishes. They tell themselves what they want and think it's enough to get there and keep them motivated. A classic example of this is New Year's. Every year, about 40% of Americans will set a resolution for the new year. Nearly 80% of those individuals will give up or fail within the first five months– some within the first three months!

A survey conducted in 2023 looked at the attitudes of Americans surrounding New Year's resolutions and what types of goals were prioritized. The most common resolutions were health-related with people saying things like:

"I want to lose weight."
"I want to eat better."
"I want to be healthier."
"I want to improve my mental health."
"I want to improve my fitness."

There's absolutely nothing wrong with wanting any of those things, but if you look closely you'll notice that none of those goals are describing anything specific. There are more than a thousand ways to achieve any one of these resolutions however, the real question is which way is going to be the one that works best for you?

For example, if your goal is to "eat better", what does that look like? Does that mean stop eating junk food and eat less calories? What about "improving mental health"? What does that mean? Meditate three times a day and stay away from politics and social media?

When it comes to weight loss, where do you start? How much weight do you want to lose? Why that amount? What routine will you follow when you wake up? How many calories will you be eating a day for *safe* weight loss? What will you eat in the morning? What will you have planned for lunch and dinner? What times will you work out at the gym? How long will you be at the gym? What exercises will you do once you're at the gym? How many days per week will you do those exercises? When will you increase or decrease the difficulty of the workout? When will you know it's the right time to change things up? I can keep going with the questioning, but hopefully you get the point.

Your goal, especially your weight loss and overall fitness, should not be vague. If it is, you'll fall into the setbacks mentioned in Chapter 1 and end up lost, confused, and frustrated like Alice in Wonderland.

In order to get to a specific destination (i.e: your desired weight loss and fit body goal), you need a specific path to follow. A well-defined goal doesn't just point you in a direction; it tells your brain what to prioritize, what to filter out, and what to ignore. In terms of brain activity, this happens through something called the **Reticular Activating System (RAS)**. It's the part of your brain that scans for what you tell it is important.

For example, that's why after you buy a new car, you suddenly see that car everywhere. That same car has been on the road the whole time, but the difference is now your brain is paying more attention to it because the car is important to you.

Your health works the same way.

As soon as you define what matters, your focus becomes stronger. You begin finding ways to act in alignment with your goal. You start seeing obstacles as signs that tell you something needs to change. We'll discuss how and when to make those changes in Chapter 10, but for now, let's create your well-defined goal to put you on the right path.

## Create a S.M.A.R.T Goal

One of the most effective tools that could help you reach your goal is what we call the SMART Goal framework. There are many different versions of this framework out there, however the one that we're going to use is adopted from Charlie Gilkey, a productivity expert, because I believe that in the context of weight loss, his version will be more effective for you.

SMART is an acronym that stands for ***specific***, ***meaningful***, ***attainable***, ***realistic***, and ***trackable***. Your goal should have all five of these elements if you want to see results fast and make them last. Here's the breakdown:

**S – Specific:** A goal is specific when you know exactly what you're aiming for. Your brain needs a target, not vague ideas. That includes giving yourself a deadline. Even if this is a lifestyle change, there should be certain milestones within your goal that you look forward to achieving within a certain time frame.

Example: *"I want to lose 15 lbs. within the next 3 months."*

**M – Meaningful:** A goal is meaningful when you know why it's important to you and how it will affect other areas in your life. This is where you find true motivation to not only achieve your goal, but also make it last. Your Fit Body goal is more than just a number on the scale.

Example: *"Losing that weight will take the pain and pressure off my knees so that I can play and run after my children without limping."*

**A – Actionable:** A goal is actionable when you know what steps you need to take or tasks to complete. Your brain needs to know which behaviors to adopt that will get you closer to your desired outcome. This also prevents you from wasting time doing things that could distract you from the big picture.

Example: *"To lose weight, I'm going to start doing some full body resistance training at least 3x a week and track my calories"*

**R – Realistic:** A goal is realistic if you're able to take action on it with the resources you currently have available. Do the best you can with what you have instead of focusing on the things that you lack.

Example: *"I have a gym membership but if I can't make it, at least I have weights at home that I can use for a full body workout."*

**T – Trackable:** A goal is trackable if there's a tangible way for you to measure progress. Tracking your results makes it easier to adjust certain behaviors so you can stay on track.

Example: *"I'm going to weigh myself every Monday with the scale I have at home. I'll record my progress in my fitness app and as a backup I'll write everything down in my fitness journal."*

## Now, It's Your Turn...

Take a moment and write down your goal using the SMART Goal framework. It's alright if you can't answer every question right now. All you're trying to do here is get clarity on your fitness goal.

> ***Specific:*** What is your fitness goal and when are you hoping to achieve it?
>
> _____
>
> ***Meaningful:*** In what ways will reaching this goal affect your life positively?
>
> _____
>
> ***Actionable:*** What are the top three things you would need to do each day in order to get you one step closer to your goal?
>
> _____
>
> ***Realistic:*** What resources do you currently have available to help you reach your goal?
>
> _____
>
> ***Trackable:*** What tools will you use and how often will you track your progress?
>
> _____

As a side note, there are two things you should consider when coming up with you own SMART Goal: pain and plateaus. Pain is a discomforting signal telling you that either something is changing or needs to change. When pain presents itself, you have two choices: you can be proactive about correcting the problem to fix the pain, or you can be reactive and let the pain make the changes for you.

If you're currently dealing with an injury or you've had a pre-existing injury that went unresolved or ignored, your first step should be to seek the proper medical professional that's best equipped to help. The kind of professional I would recommend to address your pain would be a physical therapist.

One of last things you want to do is disregard or downplay any signs that cause you pain, because this can lead to new injuries or re-injuries that will set you back. This will then lead you to be inconsistent with your workouts, which then leads to lack of results, which will ultimately lead to you quitting altogether.

Now, while pain can cause interruptions in your plan, plateaus need disruption for you to push forward.

A plateau is a point you experience when progress seems to either come really slowly or stays stagnant for a while. For instance, if at the beginning of your fitness journey you were losing about 3 pounds per week, a plateau might be that you lose half a pound every other week instead. Plateau's can make you feel as if your program isn't working or that you've reached your limit, when in actuality it's you're body telling you that it's time to change things up again.

## The Healthy Impact

I've said this before but I believe it's worth repeating: Your fit body goal is more than just a number on a scale, it's the impact that comes from pursuing your goal.

Maybe it's confidence. Maybe it's energy. Maybe it's longevity. Maybe it's showing up better for your spouse, your kids, your friends, your community, your job, or your business. Maybe it's just looking in the mirror and actually liking what you see.

Too often as I'm helping my clients reach their goals, they tend to get excited because they're seeing how pursuing their fitness goals are positively affecting other areas in their life that they hadn't considered before. And when that happens, it's like a motivation recharge that pushes them to keep going.

When your goal has meaning, it ensures that you won't quit, even during times when the number on the scale hardly changes and progress feels slow. Without something meaningful or impactful, your fitness goal will feel like a chore where you just go through the motions until eventually you lose motivation and give up.

## How Focus Prevents Setbacks

Focusing on your SMART goal not only helps you experience breakthroughs, but it better equips you to overcome barriers and prevents you from falling into the seven setbacks outlined in the beginning of this book. Here's how:

**Poor planning** is the result of not having a clearly defined goal. More importantly, poor plans are short-sighted, unpredictable, and not in alignment with your overall lifestyle, which drains your motivation and gets you inconsistent results. Your SMART goal turns confusion into clarity and points you in the direction that closely aligns your fitness goals with your overall lifestyle.

**Inconsistency** is a result of not prioritizing your health-related activities and not protecting your schedule. This opens the door for old habits and distractions to keep you stuck and prevents healthy habits from being fully formed. Focus means you commit to certain actions each day that gets you a win and allows you to get one step closer to reaching your goal.

**Tension** is stress. Too much stress creates an environment that can disrupt you hormonally, which makes it hard for you to lose weight and keep it off. Focus gives your goal structure, which can help to reduce mental overwhelm and allow you the space to find balance in other areas in your life.

A **fixed mindset** is the result of limiting beliefs that lowers confidence in your current ability to succeed based on past experiences or failures. Your SMART goal helps you reframe your focus and enables you to take action on the things that you *can* control instead of giving power to the things that you can't control.

**Adaptation** is a process that requires change. Most people quit before they reach pivotal milestones because of impatience and false expectations. Progress takes time and if you lack the commitment to make meaningful lifestyle changes, your short-term adaptations can ruin your long-term transformation. Your SMART goal prepares you for lifestyle change and allows you to realistically manage your expectations

**Lack of accountability** means no encouragement, support, or correction for when you make a mistake or feel like giving up. Your goal sets the foundation for your support system so that they can help reinforce the healthy habits and behaviors you're trying to establish. This becomes very important in the next chapter.

**Lack of dietary alignment** is the result of poor food choices and following diet plans based on unsustainable trends or severe calorie restrictions. This keeps you in an endless cycle of rapid weight loss followed by rapid weight gain, which over a long enough period, can slow down your metabolism and make it even harder to lose weight as you get older. Your SMART goal helps you focus on foods that align with your desired lifestyle and promote longevity.

## Your Focus Is Your Filter

This is why sharpening your focus changes everything. It makes the path visible, the process manageable, and makes every step towards achieving your goal more meaningful. When your focus is clear, decision-making becomes easier.

When you question whether you should skip a workout you can ask yourself, "Does this serve my goal?" When you consider grabbing takeout instead of preparing food at home, you can ask yourself, "Does this align with the plan?". In short, your focus becomes a "yes-or-no" tool that filters out distractions so that you can spend more time and energy doing things that will keep you on course.

> **Key Takeaways:**
>
> - Vague goals lead to vague results. Your fitness goal isn't a wish—it's a specific destination you're trying to reach.
>
> - Remember the SMART Goal Framework: **S**pecific, **M**eaningful, **A**ctionable, **R**ealistic, and **T**rackable
>
> - When your goal impacts more than just your weight loss, it will help motivate you to keep going.
>
> - Your focus is a filter that can prevent setbacks and allow decision-making to become easier.

Now that you have clarity on your fitness goal, the next step is to make sure nothing gets in the way of it. Focus may give you the direction, but boundaries protect that direction and accountability keeps you aligned when life inevitably challenges you. In the next chapter, we'll put guardrails around your well-defined goal so that the momentum you're creating today becomes the lifestyle you can sustain tomorrow.

\*\*\*

For quick access to resources and additional guidance for the material, scan the QR code:

## Chapter Seven

# Audit I: Boundaries & Accountability

"Your life does not get better by chance; it gets better by change."

-Jim Rohn

"The key is not to prioritize what's on your schedule, but to schedule your priorities."

-Stephen Covey

Audit is the second step within the F.A.S.T Method. It's where we put your plan in motion and create a system that allows the space for your healthy habits to thrive. If focus is the destination you plug into your GPS, then audits are the directions that take you there.

## Why You Need to Control Your Environment

If you look back to your previous weight loss attempts, I can guarantee that you would be able to spot multiple situations where life got the best of you and your program fell apart. It was usually because:

- Your schedule got hijacked

- Stress from home or work pulled you away from routine

- Your friends, family, and coworkers weren't on the same page

- You kept unhealthy foods and snacks within arms reach

- You tried to rely on willpower instead of structure

- You had no one to check in with about your progress

- You tried to "do it alone" again, even though it hasn't worked before

Practically, every single one of these is related to your environment. Your weight loss is tied to your habits and, whether you realize it or not, your habits are tied to your environment. Research has shown that roughly 40 to 50% of our daily habits are automatic, not conscious. This means, we do them because our environment nudges us to do them.

Therefore, if your environment is aligned with your health goals, then the healthy decision becomes the easy decision. But if your environment is misaligned, the unhealthy decision becomes the default. This is why we use the system I'm about to teach you called "The 3A's" to help you take back control of your environment.

## Don't Enforce an Environment You Can't Keep

Now, when it comes to taking back control of your environment, I don't want you to go overboard. Do you remember The "Biggest Loser" Study we looked at in Chapter 3? Although the contestants were in a controlled environment that supported weight loss during the show, it was extremely difficult for each of them to maintain that lifestyle in the real world.

They were constantly surrounded by celebrity coaches, trainers, and doctors; Their diet was extremely low-calorie and medically supervised; They worked out six days a week for multiple hours each day at moderate to high intensity.

Almost no one has that level of access to those kinds of resources or pushes themselves to those extremes on a regular basis, so don't try to model your environment after that. Your body doesn't see that kind of environment as sustainable or realistic.

## The 3-A's of Auditing

The 3A's stand for: **Analyze**, **Align**, and **Actualize**. It's a simple but powerful process that takes you from identifying possible problem areas within your environment to creating action steps that allow your healthy habits to feel easy and natural.

*Analyze* — This is where you take a thorough look at your environment and scan for anything that you feel either positively or negatively influences your habits. You're looking at your physical environment or spaces such as your home, work or office, places you typically shop, etc. You're also going to look at your social environment such as family, friends, coworkers, acquaintances, clubs or community.

*Align* — This is where you get to decide what stays, what changes, and what goes. The goal here is to maximize your exposure to the places, people, or things that support your goal and to minimize or eliminate everything else that goes against it.

*Actualize* — This is where you turn your decisions into simple, friction-free action steps that allow your healthy habits to become easier and make it harder for your unhealthy habits or influences to disrupt your progress.

You will use this same system again when we talk about auditing your diet and the next chapter, but here, we're going to apply it to your boundaries and accountability.

## Boundaries: Protecting Your Time, Energy, and Priorities

When people hear the word "boundaries", they sometimes think about confrontation or limitations that you set for yourself and for others. However, in the context of health and fitness, the boundaries we're talking about aren't rules we're making for others, they are about creating structure for you.

Boundaries are the commitments that protect the lifestyle you're building. The biggest boundary you want to protect and control is…your schedule.

Your schedule is the gatekeeper of your success. Your time is either managed intentionally or managed by someone else's priorities. If you don't proactively guard space for your workouts, meal prep, sleep, and recovery, the world will fill that space with distractions, requests, and friction.

## Analyze Your Time & Environment

Here are some questions to ask yourself that can help you analyze the boundary side of your time and your environment:

- What does your weekly schedule actually look like?
- Where does most of your time get spent?

- What activities drain you the most?

- What activities do you feel support your health the most?

- What current habits or relationships consistently pull you off track?

- What parts of your home or workplace encourage overeating, skipping workouts, or staying sedentary?

- What parts of your environment encourage movement, rest, productivity, or healthy food choices?

This isn't about judging anything or anyone. It's about looking at your circumstances and current situation through a realistic lens because you're not going to be able to make any *real* progress unless you do this part.

## Align Your Schedule With Your Goal

Next, you need to prioritize everything that you feel is going to support you and your goal. The mistake you want to avoid here is to tell yourself that you want to focus on your health, but you schedule says you want to:

- Be available 24/7

- Accept every invitation

- Work every overtime shift

- Watch a couple of episodes of your favorite show every night

- Handle everyone else's emergencies

Alignment here means asking questions like:

- What in my schedule actually aligns with my long-term lifestyle goal?

- What *doesn't* align even, if it's normal or feels comfortable?

- What needs to shift so my goals actually fit into my week?

- What can I eliminate or replace?

- Keep this in mind: alignment isn't about "doing more", it's about "doing what matters".

## Actualize Through Positive Stimulus Control

Now, let's put alignment into action. The key here is stimulus control, which involves changing your environment to make the desired behavior and habits easier and make the undesired behaviors harder. Here are a few examples of what this looks like:

- Scheduling your workouts at the same time every week

- Laying out your workout clothes the night before

- Blocking out specific times for other fitness-related activities

- Setting your phone to "do not disturb" during your scheduled fitness activities

- Having a "wind-down" alarm in order to mentally prepare you for sleep

Actualizing your boundary plan means literally reshaping the physical and social space around you so that the healthy choice becomes the obvious choice.

## Accountability: Your Reinforcement System

Boundaries protect your time, but accountability protects your follow-through. The research clearly shows that people with strong accountability or support systems are up to five times more likely to reach their goals! This is because accountability is what keeps you honest, consistent, and connected to your goal even when your motivation isn't at 100%.

Part of the power of accountability, is knowing what you specifically need it for. As a coach, I hold my clients accountable for the goals they set for themselves. You would expect that my clients would need constant, daily advice from me so that they stay on track, but that is rarely the case. There are some clients who seek my help with establishing healthy habits and staying on top of their routines. Then there are those clients who seek me out simply because they need someone to show up for in their calendar! In other words, they know exactly what they should be doing, but only trust they'll get it done when there is an appointment to look forward to.

Point is, we are wired for community, connection, feedback, and reinforcement. When you feel supported, it's easier for you to stay aligned. But when you're isolated, whether by choice or circumstance, you tend to drift. So, let's apply it the 3A's here:

## Analyze Your Social Influences

This part's going to feel uncomfortable but remember we're not judging anyone, we're just keeping it real with ourselves. This is where you ask yourself:

- Who in my life supports my health goals?
- Who encourages, inspires, or reinforces positive habits?
- Who consistently and distracts me or derails my efforts?
- Who pressures me into choices that conflict with my goals?
- Who do I hide my goals from because of judgment or discomfort?
- Who *actually* holds me accountable with honest feedback and who do I feel just "goes along with everything"?

People in your life will have different health priorities than you and that's to be expected. The goal is to find the people who are on the same page as we are and increase our exposure to them because there's an increased likelihood that they will keep us on track.

## Align Your Social Environment With Your Goal

Now you need to decide:

- Who do I want closer to me while I'm on my journey?
- Who can I ask for more support?
- Who do I need to communicate new boundaries with?
- Who do I need to create more space from—not to reject completely, but to protect my goals?
- What community of people, club, or group can I tap into that shares similar goals to me or has achieved the results I'm looking for?
- What accountability system matches my personality?

## Actualize Your Accountability Plan

Create a feedback and social structures for you to be supported. This can include:

*Personal accountability systems:*

- Workout journals

- Fitness apps

- Habit trackers

- Wearable technology

*Relational accountability:*

- A close friend or family member to check in with weekly

- A coworker who also wants to get healthier

- The usual members you connect with at the gym regularly

- A FaceBook group, WhatsApp, Skool group, etc.

*Professional accountability:*

- Health Coach

- Registered Dietitian or Nutritionist

- Physical Therapist

- Personal Trainer

Actualization here is about putting support around your goal so that it makes it harder to drift from it and if you do, you have guardrails to nudge you back on track. Also keep in mind that accountability isn't about control— it's about reinforcement and strengthening behaviors you've already decided to adopt.

## Reflection

*Analyze:* What **2-3 things** in your environment currently work against your goals?

*Align:* What **2-3 boundaries** or shifts would help create a healthier environment and better alignment?

*Actualize:* What **2-3 actions** can you take within the next **24 to 48 hours** to strengthen your environment and accountability?

Small actions done consistently can build big momentum. Focus on prioritizing your health habits and creating a sustainable environment that will allow you keep that momentum towards your fitness goals.

> **Key Takeaways:**
>
> - Make your environment support your health goals and healthy decisions become easier to make.
>
> - Remember the 3A's: analyze, align, and actualize.
>
> - Look at your environment carefully–without judgment, make space for things that support your goal and remove or reduce the things that don't, and take small actionable steps to bring everything in alignment.
>
> - Boundaries protect your time, but accountability protects your follow-through.

Now that you analyzed, aligned with actualized your environment, boundaries, and accountability, it's time to apply the same system to the foods you eat everyday. Your dietary environment is the most powerful element in your weight loss efforts and most people don't properly audit it.

In the next chapter, you will use the same framework to identify the foods that help you burn fat, reduce hunger, stabilize hormones, and support long-term results.

\*\*\*

For quick access to resources and additional guidance for the material, scan the QR code:

## Chapter Eight
# Audit II: Diet & Nutrition

> "Eat real food. Mostly plants. Not too much."
> -Michael Pollan

By now, you've already done something most people never do: You didn't just set a goal. You didn't just "decide" to eat better. You didn't rely on pure motivation or willpower. You took control of your schedule, your boundaries, and your accountability so that your life could start working *with* you instead of against you. Now we're going to do the same thing with food because if your physical environment affects your habits, then your dietary environment affects your body.

Most of your weight-loss efforts will break down here not because you don't care, or because you're lazy, but because your diet is completely misaligned with your desired lifestyle and it's misaligned with how sustainable fat loss *actually* works.

## Why Diet Alignment Matters More Than Calories Alone

When your diet is misaligned, it creates constant hunger, energy crashes, mood swings, stress eating, loss of control, short-term results followed by rebound weight gain. That's not an issue of you eating too few or too many calories. It's more than likely a diet alignment issue.

As we briefly talked about Part I, the problem with focusing only on calories is that you tend to ignore the content of where those calories come from. You're incentivized to eat whatever you want as long as it's within your "calorie limit" and at the same time you become desensitized to how your body responds to those foods. Even if you reduce calorie intake, the content that makes up the food (i.e. protein, fiber, water, etc.) still has an effect on leptin signals and other hunger-related hormones that will force your body to respond by telling your brain to eat more.[1]

If you haven't spent enough time establishing a new and sustainable caloric baseline through physical exercise and sensible eating patterns, your body will see calorie-restricted eating as an attack on what is considered "normal" behavior for you and respond by making weight loss difficult. This is why studies have shown that being *aware* of the calories you eat is a more effective than just counting them[2] because you're considering the overall impact the food will have on your health rather than the short-term weight loss that come from simply eating less food.

Diet alignment is about you eating in a way that is not only sustainable, but aligned with a lifestyle that has positive effects on your overall health for years to come. So, instead of me telling you what to "cut out" or "avoid", we're going to audit your diet and nutrition using the same system you just learned in the previous chapter to remove confusion and set you up for sustainable fat loss and not just short-term relief:

**Analyze → Align → Actualize**

## The 3-A's of Auditing Your Diet & Nutrition

### Analyze Your Current Diet

Before you can improve your nutrition, you need clarity. This step is about awareness, not judgment. You need to take a thorough and honest look at your dietary situation and examine, from multiple angles, which factors are affecting your food decisions. Ask yourself this:

- What do I typically eat on a normal weekday?

- What do I eat when I'm stressed, rushed, or tired?

- What foods leave me feeling full and energized?

- What foods trigger cravings, overeating, or crashes?

- How often am I relying on convenience foods?

- How often do I skip meals or under-eat early in the day?

- How often do I "save calories" only to overeat later?

- How consistent is my eating pattern week to week?


Through my experience helping my clients monitor their food choices, nearly 95% of my clients discover that most of their diet is fat dominant, meaning fat intake is well over the RDI upper limit of 35%. I have seen very few clients overdo it in both carbs and fat. Here's a simple exercise for you to try so that you can see for yourself what kind of eating pattern you're following:


## Steps to Determine Nutrient Distribution & Calorie Intake

1. ***Do a 3-Day, 5-Day, or 7-Day Food Log:*** Take some time to get a picture of what your normal eating habits are like before you try to change things ups. Three days is not a long time to get a more accurate picture, but it gives you something. In my experience, some people seem to have more patience with a shorter timeframe than the 7-Day log, however the longer you spend tracking your food for this experiment then the more accurate a picture you'll get. Your goal is to take note of EVERYTHING! Leave out no details. We're

trying to be honest with ourselves about our diet.

2. ***Figure out Your Total Daily Energy Expenditure (TDEE):*** There are plenty of apps and tools online to do this math for you, but essentially you want to figure out how much total energy your body uses in a given day.

3. ***Determine Ideal Caloric Intake:*** This is where you take the TDEE from Step 1, and determine what you want your daily calorie goal to be. TDEE represents how many calories it would take for you to maintain your current situation. For example, if your TDEE says you currently burn 2,000 calories a day, then in order to maintain, you would need to consume at least 2,000 calories to keep everything the same. Since we're focused on weight loss, what you want to do then is take the TDEE and subtract 500 calories and that would give you a rough sense of how many calories you would need to consume in order to burn about 1 pound of fat per week. Using the same example above, you would then aim to consume 1,500 calories instead of 2,000. (Note: Generally speaking, they say that 1 pound of fat equals about 3,500 calories. 500 calories x 7 days/week = 3,500 calories or 1 pound of fat)

4. ***Determine Macronutrient Distribution:*** This is where you get to see where all of those calories are coming from. I like the idea that 15 – 25% of your caloric intake should come from protein, 25% or less calories should come from fats, and 50 – 60% from carbohydrates. Later on, we'll talk more about why that suggested ratio for weight loss, but essentially this is where we break down how many calories are

coming from which macronutrients (i.e: proteins, fats, carbohydrates). After you do this, make a comparison between how your current diet lines up with the suggested ratios.

Most people already *know* which foods work against them. The problem is that they just haven't connected those foods to lack of fat loss, chronic hunger, stress, and even inflammation.

## Align With the Universal Principle of Successful Diets

We've discussed the five components that make any diet successful for long-term weight loss and maintenance back in Chapter 4. In this step, we're going to put those components together and I'm going to give you my formula to help you choose the best foods to align with your goals. Just to recap, remember that **longevity is lean.** The food components that are associated with longevity are also associated with helping you stay lean.

## The Fit Body F.A.S.T Food Formula

Here's the formula:
1. Focus on fiber

2. Eat lean protein

3. Eat less fat

4. Drink more water

## Focus on Fiber (The 4 F's of Fiber)

Fiber is known for four things: fullness, frequency, fuel, and fat loss. We know that fiber can create a feeling of fullness by slowing down the time it takes for food to leave the stomach, which can help with appetite suppression and overall lower caloric intake.[3] With lower overall caloric intake from fiber, you can also experience gradual weight loss over time. [4,5]

Frequency or regular bowel movement, on the other hand, doesn't get talked about enough when discussing diet. If you're experiencing irregular bowel movement, then adding fiber can help with regularity. This is really important because if stool sits in your gut for too long, it can cause abdominal pain, constipation, and it can even start to produce toxins that get reabsorbed back into your bloodstream and have negative effects on your kidneys and immune system.[6] You want to avoid having that kind of gut problem as much as possible by maintaining regular bowel movement, which can range anywhere from three times per day to three days per week depending on the person.

Dietary fiber can *only* be found in plant sources. The best sources of fiber includes: berries (strawberries, blackberries, blueberries, cherries, raspberries, etc.), other fruits (apple, banana, orange, mango, avocado, plum, pear, kiwi, etc.), legumes (black beans, pinto beans, kidney beans, chickpeas, lentils, etc.), grains (brown rice, quinoa, oats, buckwheat, spelt, etc.), vegetables (broccoli, spinach, carrots, potatoes, sweet potatoes, yucca, brussel sprouts, cabbage, kale, beets, etc.), nuts and seeds (almonds, cashews, pistachios, chestnuts, Brazil nuts, chia seeds, flax seeds, pumpkin seeds, sunflower seeds, etc.).

Fruits typically have anywhere from 2g-8g per serving, legumes will have 6g-8g per ½ cup, grains will have 2g-6g per serving (try to go for a ratio of 1g of fiber for every 10g or less of carbohydrates), vegetables will have roughly 2g-6g per ½ cup and sometimes up to 7g per cup, nuts will have 1g-4g per ounce (or about a handful), and seeds will have anywhere from 3g-10g per tablespoon.

The average person only consumes about 15g of fiber per day, however the optimal range for fiber intake for adult men is 35g and 25g for adult women. If you play around with a variety of different fruits and vegetables, you will most likely get in all the fiber you need. But if you're not used to eating that much fiber, start with what you feel your body can currently tolerate and work from there.

## Eat Lean Protein

According to the Food and Nutrition Board, who set the Recommended Daily Allowance (RDA) to determine what is sufficient to meet nutrient requirements, states that the goal for daily protein intake is 0.8g/kg of bodyweight or 0.36g/lb of body weight if you're a more sedentary individual. If you're more active, then 1.2g/kg of bodyweight or 0.6g/lb of body weight is recommended.

To give you an idea: as a 170 lb male (or 77.27 kg), I would need to consume 61.2g of protein (170 x 0.36) on the low end and 102g of protein on the "high" end (170 x 0.6). You have probably heard that you need to eat at least 1g per 1 pound of protein for your body weight, but I believe that can be a bit excessive for most people. Although there is good evidence that shows significant weight loss with high protein consumption[7], in my experience, the RDA recommendations work fine and it's very attainable to get that much protein through food.

They say that 10% to 35% of your calories should come from protein as well. Personally, I like the 15% to 25% sweet spot for protein. For example, most dieters would probably eat around 1,500 kcal. This would mean that about 94g of protein would be your goal (1,500 x 0.25 = 375. Then 375/4 = 93.75).

Lastly, you want to make sure the protein is "lean". The United States Department of Agriculture (USDA) considers a protein source as "lean" if it contains less than 10g of total fat (less than 4.5g of saturated fat) and less than 93 milligrams of cholesterol per 100g (i.e: 3.5 oz) serving. Put another way, for every ounce of a protein source there should be 3g or less of fat.

According to the USDA's definition, plant proteins are the *leanest* form of proteins you can find because they naturally come with very little fat, if any, per gram or ounce of protein. Lentils, beans, tofu, edamame, oats, chia seeds, are just a few plant sources that come to mind when we're talking about high amounts of protein with very little fat.

## Eat Less (Saturated) Fat

We covered saturated fat consumption back in Chapter 4, and we understand that overconsumption of this kind of fat can lead to weight gain as exploited by the owner of the Most Dangerous Restaurant. As a reminder, saturated fat is the kind of fat that that's usually found in sources such as fatty cuts of red meat, poultry skin, full-fat dairy, cheese, tallow, lard, butter, and even fried foods. One long-term study explored the relationship between dietary fat intake and its effect on U.S. men and women in regard to weight gain over the span of 24 years. Every four years they did a follow up with participants, in which they found that with just a 5% increase in caloric intake from saturated fats led to anywhere between 1 – 2 lbs. of weight gain.[8]

That doesn't sound like much and it's not surprising given the fact that if you just added extra calories to your diet then the obvious result should be weight gain. But what's interesting, was that researchers also found that the extra calories from unsaturated fats or polyunsaturated fats (i.e: fats typically found in nuts, seeds, avocados, etc.), wasn't associated with weight gain. These kinds of fats are actually associated with *weight decrease*. Other studies have shown that diets high in saturated fat not only is associated with bodyweight increase, but it's also associated with increased liver fat and insulin resistance.[9]

Aside from this and other evidence, it's probably a good idea of consume less than 25% of your total calories from fat (less than 10% of total calories from saturated fats is what's also recommended) and to the best of your ability, consume sources higher in monounsaturated and polyunsaturated fats.

## Drink More Water

Our bodies are made up of approximately 70 to 75% of water, so hydration is important. The average adult drinks less than 4 cups of water per day, which is far less from the adequate intake range of 15.5 cups for males and 11.5 cups for females according to the U.S. National Academies of Sciences, Engineering, and Medicine (US-NASEM).

Let's assume that you regularly consume proper servings of foods such as fruits and vegetables, then about 20% of water intake can come from that, which makes the adequate water intake roughly 12 cups per day for males and 8 cups per day for females. Regular water consumption is linked to weight loss[10], so when you're diligent about consuming adequate amounts of water regularly, it will aid in your efforts to lose weight and be fit.

## Diet Alignment Means Asking Better Questions

When those components are present, fat loss becomes easier. This is why wildly different diets can all "work" when they improve the food quality to align with longevity. The problem isn't that you can't find the "right" diet, the problem is choosing a diet you can't sustain because they don't emphasize all of these components. Sometimes, diet alignment means asking yourself better questions so that you can feel confident in making better food choices.

Instead of asking: "How fast can I lose weight?"
Ask: "How can I eat in a way I can maintain?"

Instead of asking: "What should I cut out?"
Ask: "What foods are lean in protein, provide fiber, and are low in fat, that can help me feel full and energized?"

Instead of asking: "What diet is best?"
Ask: "What eating patterns out there aligns with my life, schedule, and promotes longevity?"

Diet alignment shifts the goal from restriction and control to consistency and sustainability. Many people take a negative approach to dieting because they feel that in order for it to be enjoyable and worthwhile, there should be some kind of "cheat". Let me ask you a question: If you told your spouse that you would need one day out of the week to sleep with someone else in order to feel happy, how long would you expect that marriage to last? Probably not long. So why do we approach diet with the same attitude expecting it to be successful?

Any diet that makes you look forward to a "cheat meal" or "cheat day" will almost always be the one you can't sustain. Your diet shouldn't feel so restrictive that you crave "freedom" from it periodically.

## Actualize Into Daily Eating Habits

You probably won't have much of an issue eating well on calm days, but most of your fat loss success will depend on how you handle stressful days. If you find simple foods and come up with simple, repeatable meals to that align with the four components we just discussed, then those stressful days will slowly start to work themselves out. Start by asking yourself:

- What do I eat when I'm in a rush?

- What do I grab when I'm exhausted?

- What do I default to when I don't want to think?

## Remove Friction *Then* Adjust Foods

Most people go straight to restricting certain foods from their diet and then stress about what options are available to eat once they've cleaned out the pantry. Instead of jumping right into removing foods:

- Keep nutrient-dense foods visible and easily accessible

- Make less aligned foods harder to access

- Reduce decision-making around your meals by pre-commit to grocery lists and meal patterns

When you give yourself easier access to healthier foods first, it can become easier later to adjust and remove the other foods in your diet that aren't in alignment with your goals. Fast food restaurants use this tactic all the time and they're successful because they make access to their foods so easy and frictionless. They make every food decision too easy for you to say "yes". Let's copy their winning strategy and make it easier for you to choose the right foods instead.

> **Key Takeaways:**
>
> - Analyze your current diet to see where you might be sabotaging your efforts but also see where the opportunities are to make changes.
>
> - Align your food choices with your long-term health goals and you'll find foods that are naturally associated with weight loss.
>
> - Actualize your eating habits so that you can take control of your stressful days and eat the right foods. Don't go straight to cutting out foods, but instead remove friction from the healthy decisions that are in front of you before you cut out the bad options.
>
> - Remember the formula: 1) Eat more lean protein 2) Focus on Fiber 3) Eat less saturated fat 4) Drink more water

Now that you've audited your diet nutrition, and now that you've made it actionable, it's time to add the third piece to strengthen your weight loss and fit body results. We're going to look at exercises you can use to build a stronger body, increase your metabolism, and burn some fat.

\*\*\*

For quick access to resources and additional guidance for the material, scan the QR code:

# References

1. Benton, David, and Hayley A Young. "Reducing Calorie Intake May Not Help You Lose Body Weight." *Perspectives on psychological science : a journal of the Association for Psychological Science* vol. 12,5 (2017): 703-714. doi:10.1177/1745691617690878

2. Benton, David, and Hayley A Young. "Reducing Calorie Intake May Not Help You Lose Body Weight." *Perspectives on psychological science : a journal of the Association for Psychological Science* vol. 12,5 (2017): 708-709.

3. Salleh, Siti Nurshabani et al. "Unravelling the Effects of Soluble Dietary Fibre Supplementation on Energy Intake and Perceived Satiety in Healthy Adults: Evidence from Systematic Review and Meta-Analysis of Randomised-Controlled Trials." *Foods (Basel, Switzerland)* vol. 8,1 15. 6 Jan. 2019, doi:10.3390/foods8010015

4. Miketinas, Derek C et al. "Fiber Intake Predicts Weight Loss and Dietary Adherence in Adults Consuming Calorie-Restricted Diets: The POUNDS Lost (Preventing Overweight Using Novel Dietary Strategies) Study." *The Journal of nutrition* vol. 149,10 (2019): 1742-1748. doi:10.1093/jn/nxz117

5. Kelly, Rebecca K et al. "Increased dietary fiber is associated with weight loss among Full Plate Living program participants." *Frontiers in nutrition* vol. 10 1110748. 17 Apr. 2023,

doi:10.3389/fnut.2023.1110748

6. Johnson-Martínez, Johannes P et al. "Aberrant bowel movement frequencies coincide with increased microbe-derived blood metabolites associated with reduced organ function." *Cell reports. Medicine* vol. 5,7 (2024): 101646. doi:10.1016/j.xcrm.2024.101646

7. Moon, Jaecheol, and Gwanpyo Koh. "Clinical Evidence and Mechanisms of High-Protein Diet-Induced Weight Loss." *Journal of obesity & metabolic syndrome* vol. 29,3 (2020): 166-173. doi:10.7570/jomes20028

8. Liu, Xiaoran et al. "Changes in Types of Dietary Fats Influence Long-term Weight Change in US Women and Men." *The Journal of nutrition* vol. 148,11 (2018): 1821-1829. doi:10.1093/jn/nxy183

9. Rosqvist, Fredrik, et al. "*Overeating Saturated Fat Promotes Fatty Liver and Ceramides Compared With Polyunsaturated Fat: A Randomized Trial.*" *The Journal of Clinical Endocrinology & Metabolism*, vol. 104, no. 12, Dec. 2019, pp. 6207–6219. Oxford University Press, https://doi.org/10.1210/jc.2019-00160

10. Bracamontes-Castelo, Guillermo et al. "Effect of water consumption on weight loss: a systematic review." "Efecto del consumo de agua sobre la pérdida de peso: revisión sistemática." *Nutricion hospitalaria* vol. 36,6 (2019): 1424-1429. doi:10.20960/nh.02746

# Chapter Nine
# Strengthen

"Exercise is labour without weariness."

-Samuel Johnson

"A fit, healthy body—that is the best fashion statement."

-Jess C. Scott

Without a doubt, nutrition will be the biggest component to weight loss and fat loss. Almost everyone knows about the calories-in versus calories-out principle, but many don't seem to realize that we have way more control over the "calories-in" part than we do "calories-out". This is why if you don't get the diet part right first, it doesn't matter matter how hard you work out or whatever exercises you do. Studies have shown that exercise alone can contribute to some weight loss, but diet *plus* exercise produces significantly better results.[1]

This may sound like I'm discrediting exercise and it's impact on weight loss, but I can assure you that's not the case. I believe some movement is better than no movement at all. I just want to drive home the point that just because you feel like you're crushing it in the gym does not mean that a double cheeseburger and that slice of pizza won't ruin all of your hard work.

## Focus On Moving

The World Health Organization (WHO) recommends that adults participate in at least 150-300 minutes of moderate-intensity exercise or 75-150 minutes of high-intensity exercise per week. These seem like reasonable goals to meet but is it enough when it comes to exercising for weight loss? According to the U.S. Department of Health and Human Services Physical Activity Guidelines Advisory Committee, roughly 300 minutes of moderately intense activity per week is sufficient to at least keep your weight stable. They actually recommend that the minimum you should strive for is 450 minutes of moderate-intense exercise per week and at least half of that if you're doing high-intensity exercise.

To translate, that's about an about 1.5 hours of moderate-intense exercise and about 45 minutes of high-intensity exercise per day (if you decide to rest on the weekends). Keep in mind that when it comes to high-intensity exercise, shoot for at least three days throughout the week and mix in some moderate-intense exercise in between days. You do not want to perform high-intensity exercise every day because it can be too much on the body over the long-term.

If we follow the WHO's recommendations, we would just scratch the surface of our fat burning potential with exercise. With the latter recommendations for exercise, however, we could potentially burn anywhere from 500-850 calories per day and shed at least a half a pound to a pound per week. Couple this with a diet optimized for longevity, and you're looking at losing up to 24 pounds in as little as 12 weeks!

## 3-2-1 Cardio

When looking at the different types of exercises and their effect on blood pressure, blood sugar control, physical strength, and fat metabolism, combined training (i.e: aerobic exercise plus resistance training) was proven to be the most effective on impacting those areas in individuals who are overweight or obese.[2] With that said, aerobic (i.e: cardio) exercise can still lead to weight loss.

Anyone can take advantage of a simple exercise such as walking, especially if performed under different intensities. Research has shown that taking a brisk fifteen to thirty minute walk, especially after consuming a meal, can lower the risk of coronary heart disease, increase immune function, increase mood and energy levels, stabilize blood sugar, and help burn fat.[3,4]

One method you can use to take advantage of fat-burning effects of cardio is the "3-2-1 Cardio" approach. This approach is basically a 3-minute walk followed by a 2-minute jog followed by a 1-minute run.

You would repeat this cycle for 6-12 rounds giving you anywhere from thirty minutes to an hour of exercise.

This approach would be considered interval training and can access the "**afterburn effect**" if done after a few rounds. The "afterburn effect", also known as the state of excess post-oxygen consumption (EPOC), is where your body tends burns more calories in order to make up for the increased rate of oxygen usage during exercise. The effects of EPOC can last for hours after exercise has been completed.

This exercise approach can be done both before or after a workout session as a warmup and cooldown, if it's not too intense. You can also make this its own workout by doing it on a non-resistance training rest day where, instead of thirty minutes, you can brisk/power walk for an hour. However, if you want. to keep the intensity moderate, you can use this approach for an active rest day.

## The 4 Fundamental Strength Exercises That Build Body's & Burn Fat

Before you attempt to perform any of the exercises found in this section, please make sure to stretch and warmup properly! Spend at least 5 – 15 minutes before your workout to do a dynamic stretch and when your workout is finished, do a 5 – 15 minute cooldown and static stretch.

There are essentially four core exercises or movements your workout regimen should include for overall functional strength: squat, deadlift, bench press (or push press), and shoulder press (i.e. overhead or vertical press).

## Squats

When it comes to burning fat and building muscle, squats are amazing. One of the largest and most powerful muscle groups in the entire body are in our back and legs, which is why I started this section off with this exercises. Other than the fact that you can build significant strength and burn fat, why do this exercise at all? Simply put: because you perform the squat movement everyday. Whether you realize it or not, almost all of our daily motions and actions require us to squat. Therefore, strengthening your quads and glutes through squatting will make everyday tasks more efficient while at the same time help you lose weight.

## (Back) Squat

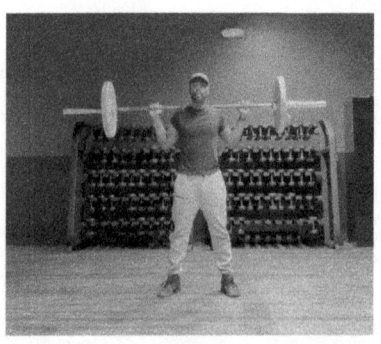

1.) Step up to the bar facing it and make sure you're centered between both ends of the bar. 2.) Step underneath the bar and grip the bar making sure that the bar is resting on rear deltoid and/or the meatier part of your upper trapezius.

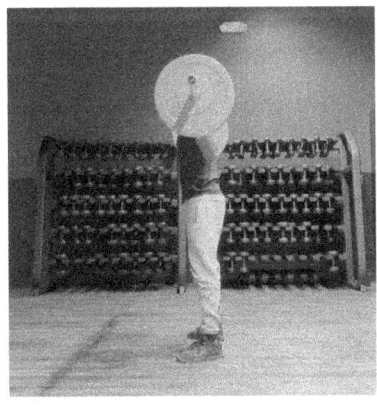

3.) Stand with feet about shoulder-width apart and toes pointed out slightly (between 10° and 30°) 4.) Before you descend into the squatted position, take a quick inhale, keep your head and chest up while keeping your abs tight.

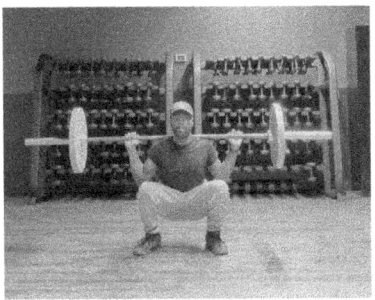

5.) As you descend, you want to break at the hips and push the glutes outward behind you. 6.) Go as low as you can while keeping your head and chest up; you also want to make sure that you're sitting back on your heels and keeping your feet flat on the ground throughout the entire exercise. If your knees start to cave in, then make an effort to push them out so that they're over your feet. However, don't force your knees too far out that the inside of your feet come up off of the ground.

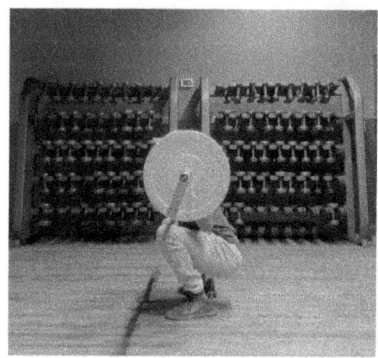

7.) Once you've reached the bottom of your squat, you're going to exhale and drive through the heels, knees and hips back into upright standing position. 8.) Make sure to squeeze the glutes once back at starting position to lock out at the hips.

## Deadlift

One of my favorite exercises is the Deadlift. Both functional and intense, this exercise can give you a huge bang for your buck in any workout regimen. This one lift alone can target glutes, lats, core and hamstrings. I myself practice three variations of this exercise that I will demonstrate below but first I must state that as awesome as this exercise is, it can be very taxing on both the nervous so make sure you warm up properly before you jump into this exercise.

## Conventional Deadlift

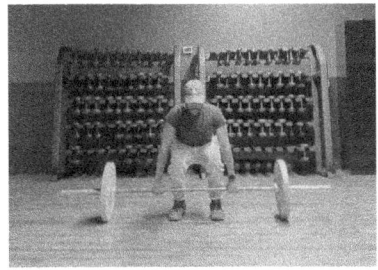

1.) Stand with feet about hip-width apart with the bar lined up directly over the center of your feet. 2.) Bend hips and knees, getting into a squat position, to grip the bar. You want your hand placement to be just outside of your legs. 3.) When gripping the bar, start with an overhand grip (both palms facing you). As you progress and weight gets heavier, you may wish to use an over-under grip or "mixed" grip (one palm facing toward you and the other facing away) for improved stability when holding the bar.

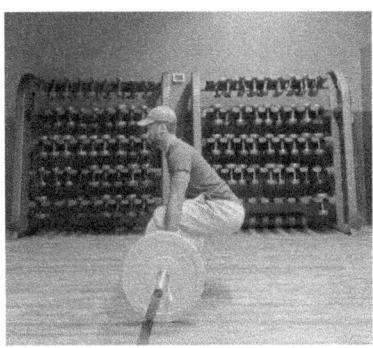

4.) Make sure your shoulders are pressed back and down. 5.) Your back should remain flat (i.e. neutral spine position), from the base of your skull to the tailbone, through the entire exercise. **Note: If you cannot keep your back flat through the entire exercise while lifting weight directly from the floor, then you can raise the platform on which you're lifting the weight. It's not cheating! The goal is to do the exercise with the best form possible.**

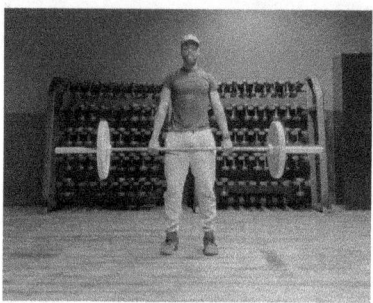

6.) When lifting and lowering, the bar should remain in contact with your legs throughout the whole motion. 7.) Make sure your knees and hips are working together to lift the weight into upright locked position and back to starting position.

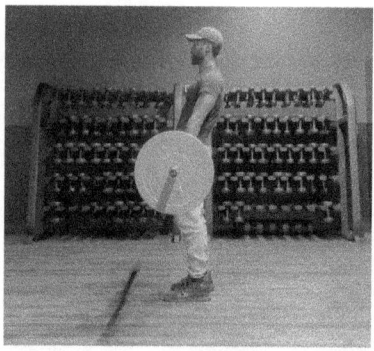

## Sumo Deadlift

Sumo Deadlift is a personal favorite of mine simply because it's very comfortable for me and I'm able to generate a great deal of power from this stance. When setting up the for Sumo Deadlift, Steps 1 and 2 will differ from both the Conventional and the Romanian.

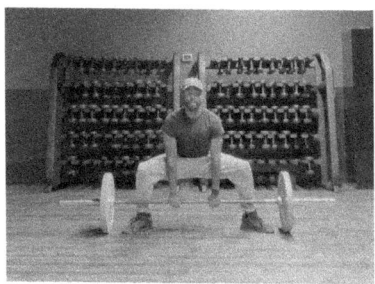

Instead of standing with your feet hip-width apart and toes facing forward, your stance will be wider (a little wider than shoulder-width) and toes pointed out anywhere between 20° to 45°. Lastly, because your stance is wider, your hand placement will be between your legs instead of right outside your knees. Try to align yourself directly in the middle of the bar and leave about ten to twelve inches of space between your hands when gripping the bar. All other steps in the Conventional Deadlift can be applied here.

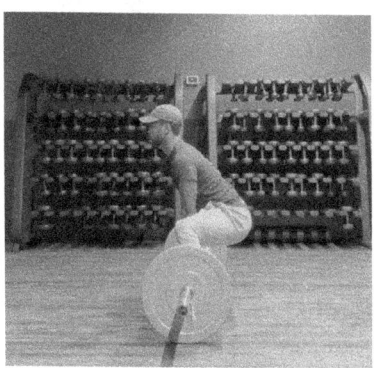

(Note: Since your stance is wider in the sumo position, your center of mass is closer to the ground, which means the weight doesn't have to travel that far from the ground to complete the lift. For this reason, some people think that this version of the deadlift makes it easier, however, the Sumo Deadlift demands more muscular contractions from your glutes, adductors, and all of the muscles that make up your pelvic floor than the Conventional deadlift.)

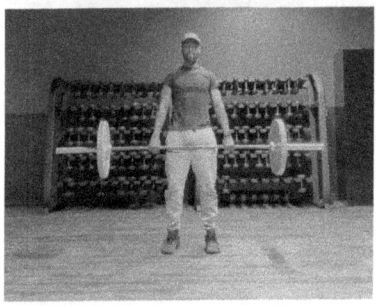

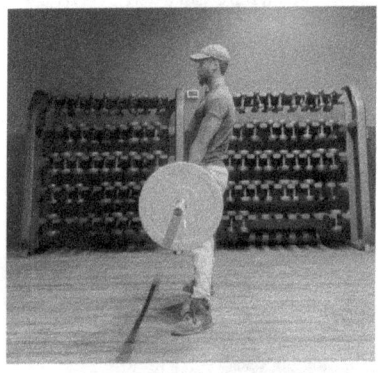

## Romanian Deadlift

As with the Sumo variation, the Romanian Deadlift will slightly differ from the Conventional in terms of set up and movement. Whereas the Conventional has a set up similar to that of a squat in Step

2, for the Romanian position you're going to keep your legs almost straight (with about a 20% bend in the knees) and bend at the hips to reach for the bar.

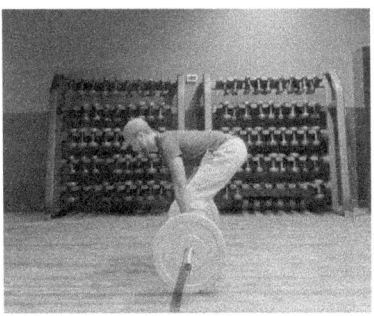

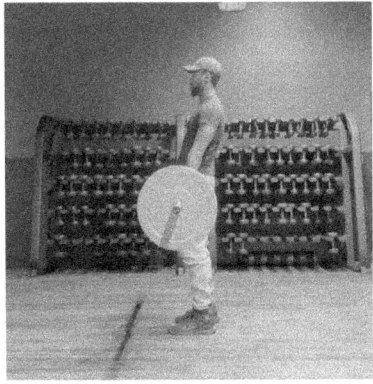

Follow Steps 3 through 6 from the Conventional variation and remember to squeeze your glutes at the top of your lift. Neutral spine position is a must throughout the entire lifting motion. This is a very glute and hamstring dominant exercise, so you want to make sure your properly warmed up prior to this lift.

# Overhead Press

This is arguably one of the best shoulder/upper body exercises aside from the bench press. The overhead press stimulates the anterior (front) shoulder muscles, triceps, back, and core. Because you're lifting the weight directly over your body, your abdominal muscles as well as your upper back muscles need to help stabilize the weight so that it doesn't fall forward or backwards.

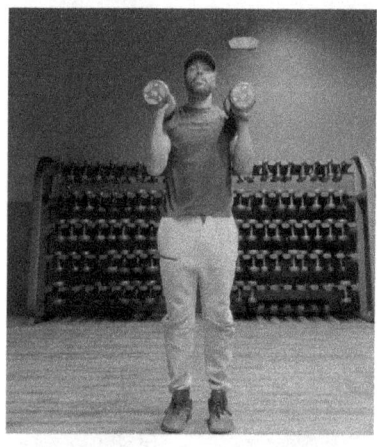

1.) Starting position requires that the bar (or dumbbells) is right above the upper chest but lower than chin level. 2.) Make sure your wrists are in locked position and directly over your elbows.

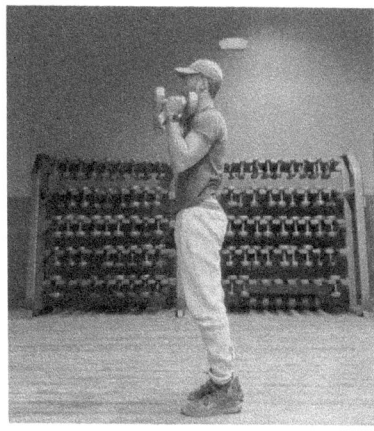

3.) Make sure your feet are about hip-width apart and that you're keeping your heels on the ground at all times. 4.) Stabilize your core and try not to arch your back as you press the weight directly above your head.

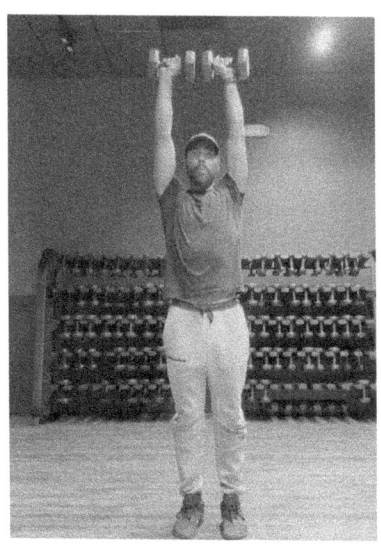

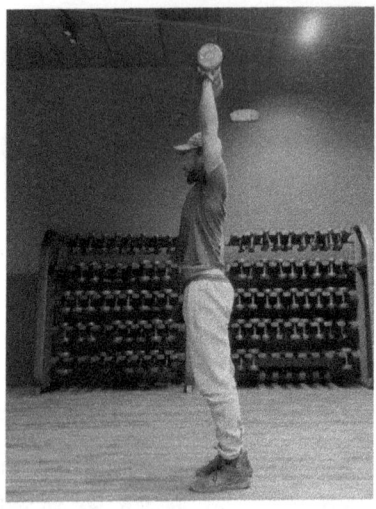

5.) Try not to look up at the weight or it can cause unwanted arching of the spine and apply unnecessary stress on the lower back.
6.) Make sure your arms are fully locked out at the top of the press before returning the weight back to starting position.

## Chest Press

This exercise is for more than just building chest muscles. You're strengthening your core, front shoulder, and triceps as well. The most common way people strengthen their chest is through the bench press, however you don't need to have a barbell or even need to perform this particular exercise to strengthen the chest. You can use dumbbells or just your bodyweight by performing the standard push up to strengthen all of those areas mentioned.

## Floor Press

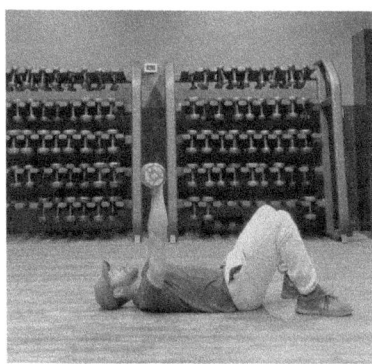

1.) Lie on your back with knees bent and feet flat.

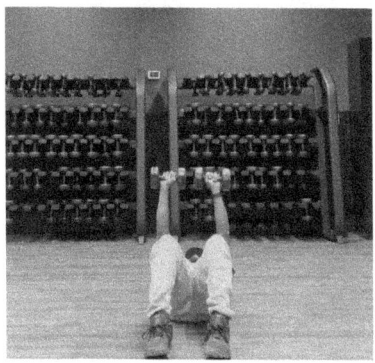

2.) Hold weights with elbows on the floor, arms bent. 3.) Press the weights straight up until your arms are straight.

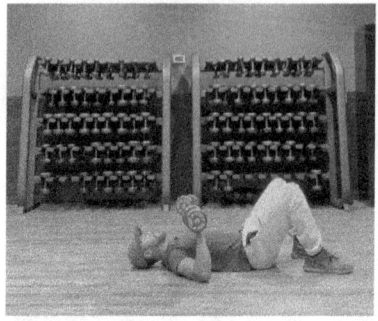

4.) Lower slowly until elbows touch the floor again.

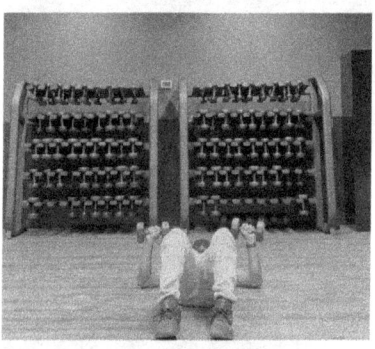

**Push-Up**

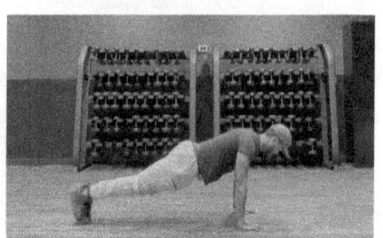

1.) Get into a plank position with arms extended, hands placed directly under the shoulders, and feet together while bracing the core.

2.) Keep your head up at about a 45 degree angle so that your eyes are fixated at a point in the ground about three to four feet in front of you.

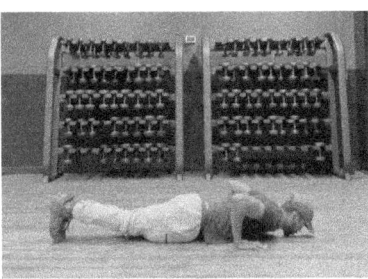

3.) Bend at the elbows dropping your chest until it touches the floor. 4.) Once your chest touches the floor, push down into the ground, lifting your chest off of the ground until you get back into the straight arm starting plank position.

## Modified Push Up Variations

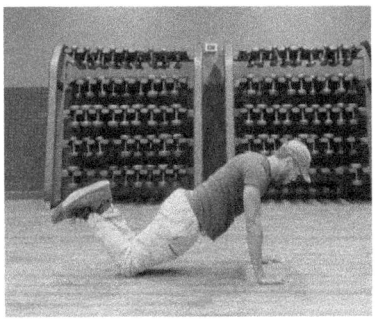

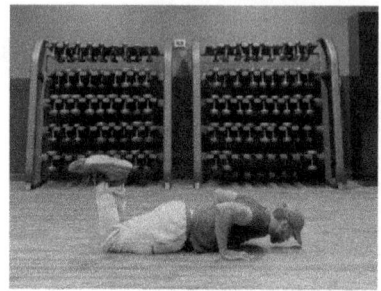

If you're not able to do a conventional push up then try the modified version. It follows the same steps and principles with the exception that instead of you having your feet extended and your toes are the point of contact with the floor, it's your knees. Another thing you can try is doing the push up from an elevated position such as on a box, chair, counter top, etc.

\*\*\*

Those are basically the four core movements that make up any solid, functional strength workout. Now, let's add onto these with some exercises I perform with some of my clients. In this next section, please don't feel like you need to have all of these exercises in your workout regimen in order to get a good workout. These are just a few selected exercises I use with clients to get them moving and give them a good workout.

## No Equipment to Low Equipment Exercises

This section is designed with a "No Excuses" approach meaning that there is no reason or excuse for you to not exercise. Believe it or not, but you have everything you need to build the body you want whether you have access to equipment or not. The exercises selected for this book are by no means the "be-all and end-all", but through research, evidence, and experience they have been proven time and time again to give you a solid workout. We're going to start with exercises easiest to implement with no equipment (i.e. bodyweight), and then build up to exercises that require minimal equipment.

## Body Weight Exercises

### Forward/Backward Lunges

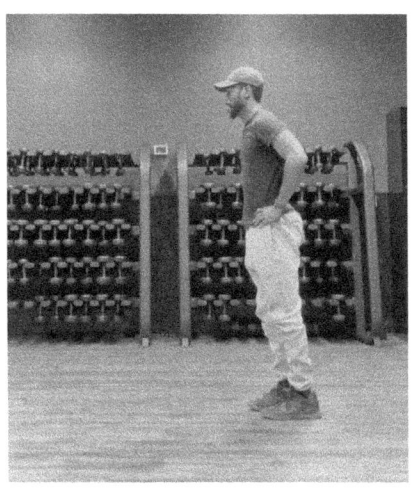

1. Stand with your feet at least hip-width apart. You can start with your hands either by side, on your hips or behind you head.

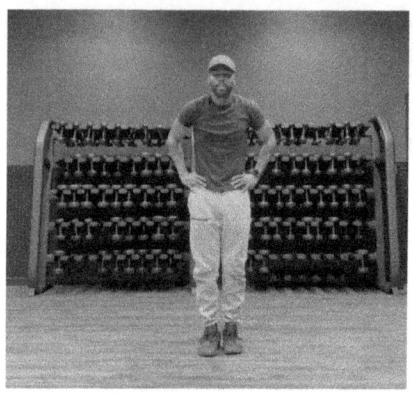

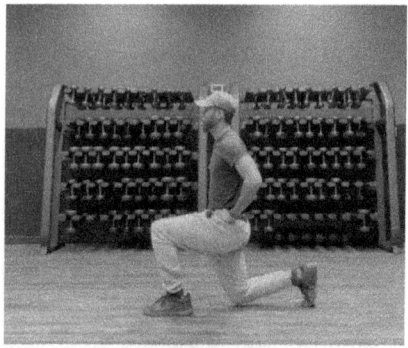

2.) Take big step forward, shifting the weight to the lunging leg, making sure heel touches the ground first. [When performing the backward lunge, you're going to take a big step backwards making sure the balls of your feet make contact with the ground]

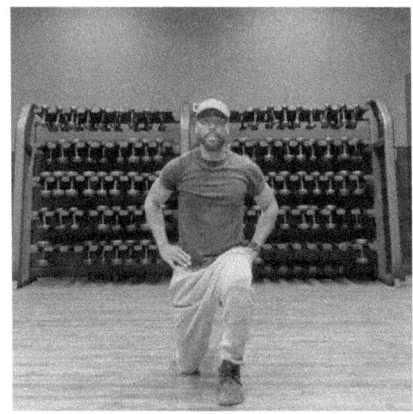

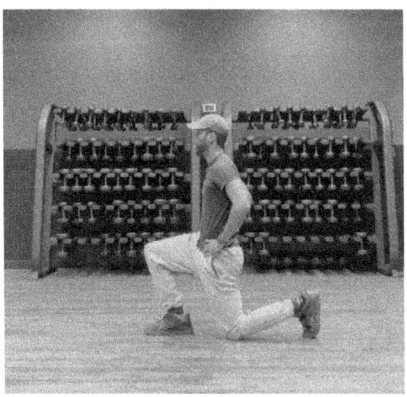

3.) Once your front foot is flat on the ground, drop the back knee as low as you can to the ground so that the forward thigh is parallel to the ground. Make sure you're keeping you chest up and back straight. [Drop the back knee down towards the ground. If you notice that your front knee is past your toes then take a bigger step backwards to adjust.] 4.) Push off of the heel of the forward leg to drive yourself back into starting position. [Push off of the back foot to drive yourself back to starting position.]

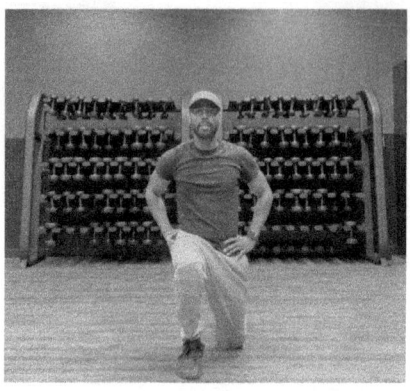

5.) Repeat the same steps with the other leg.

Note: As with the squats, you want to make sure that you're keeping your weight on your heels when you lunge. When lunging forward with the front leg, try to make sure you heel is in contact with the floor. Try not to shift your weight too far forward over your knees as this will drive your knees over your toes and force the heel off of the ground.

## Backward Lunge to High Knee Jump

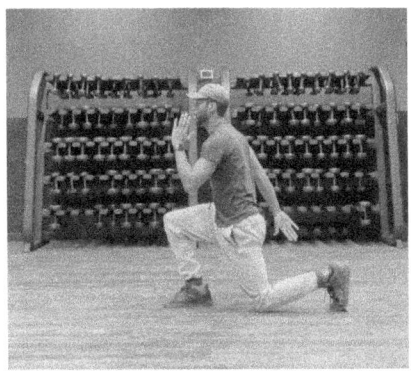

1.) Stand tall with feet hip-width apart. 2.) Step one foot straight back and bend both knees.

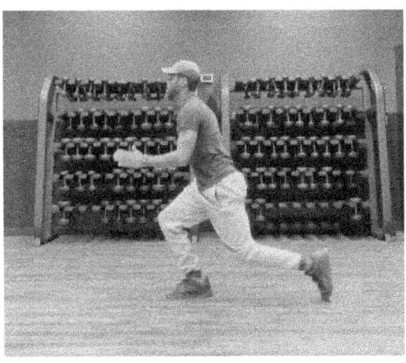

3.) Push through the front foot into a small hop.

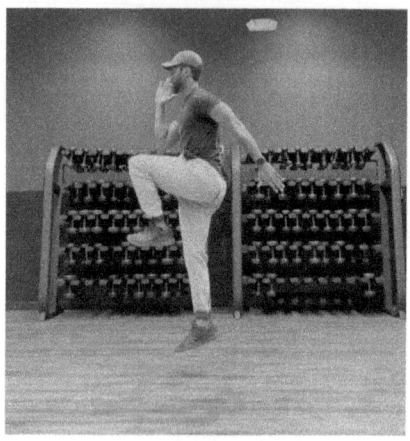

4.) As you jump up, drive the knee up toward your chest. 5.) Lower the foot and repeat, then switch sides.

## Curtsy Lunge

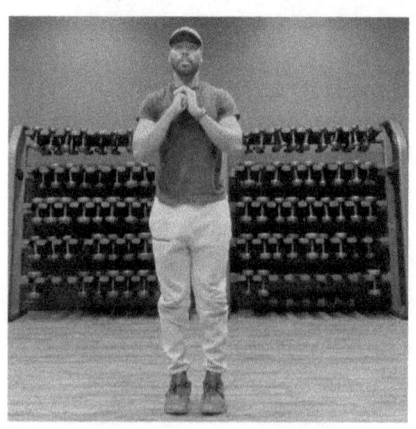

1.) Stand tall with feet around hip-width apart.

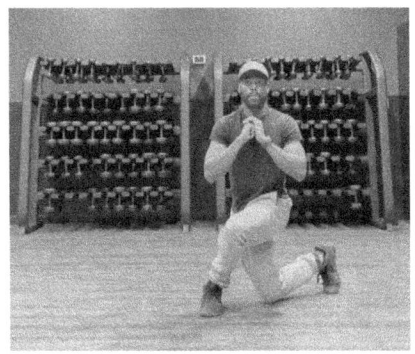

2.) Step one foot back and across behind the other leg. 3.) Bend both knees and lower your body like a small squat. 4.) Keep your chest up and knees pointing forward.

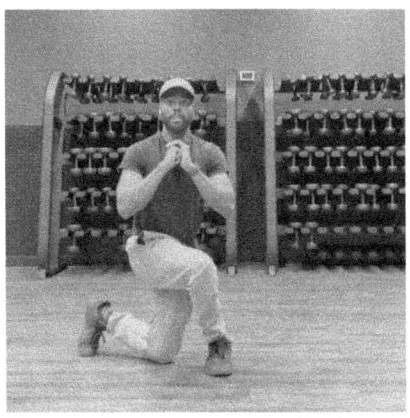

5.) Push through the front heel to stand back up. 6.) Switch legs and repeat.

## Lateral Lunges

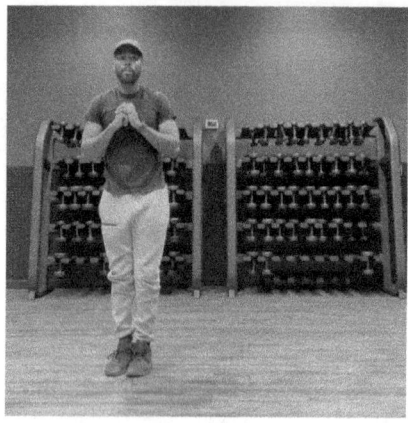

1.) Take a big lateral step to either the right or left side, shifting your weight to towards the lunging leg while keeping your head and chest up.

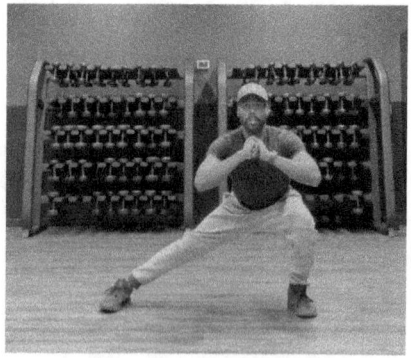

2.) Much like the squat, you're going to push your hips back and then bend at the knees. Make sure your heel stays in contact with the ground. (With the lunging leg, you may want to turn your foot outwards about 30° so that it opens up your lunge.

# THE FIT BODY F.A.S.T. METHOD 155

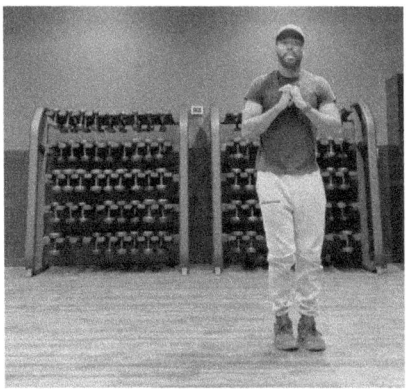

3.) Try to keep the opposite leg relatively straight and the foot flat on the ground. 4.) Push off of the lunged leg by driving off of your heels back into starting position.

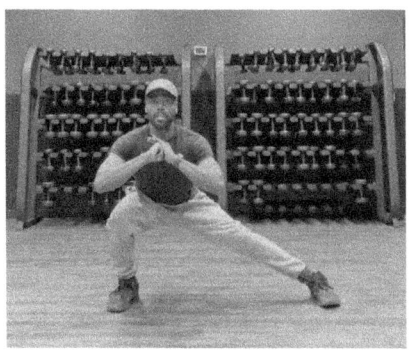

5.) Repeat the process on the opposite side.

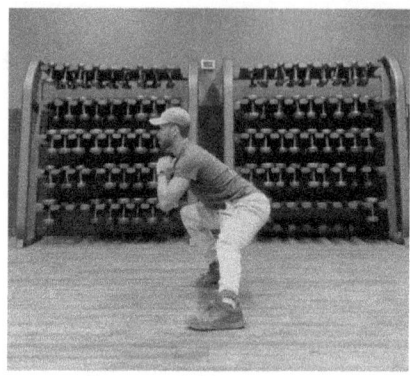

## Prisoner/ Bodyweight Squat

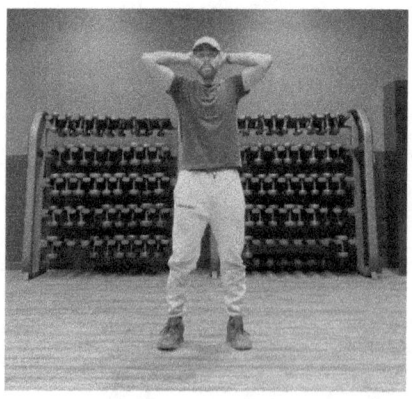

1.) Start in an upright standing position with your feet about hip-width apart. 2.) Take a nice big inhale and brace your core.

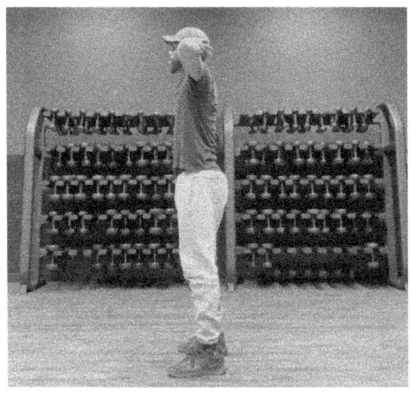

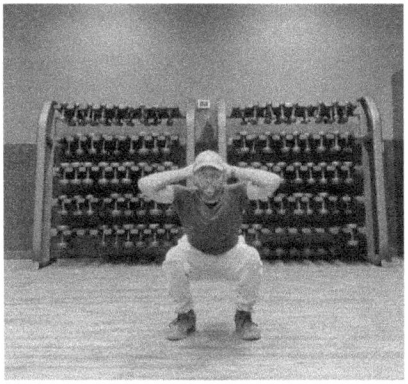

3.) Bend at the hips first (also called "hip hinging") then bend at the knees to bring your glutes and hips to the ground. You want to try get get your hips to 90 degrees or below. 4.) Make sure to keep your core engaged, your chest up, and your heels on the ground throughout the entire exercise.

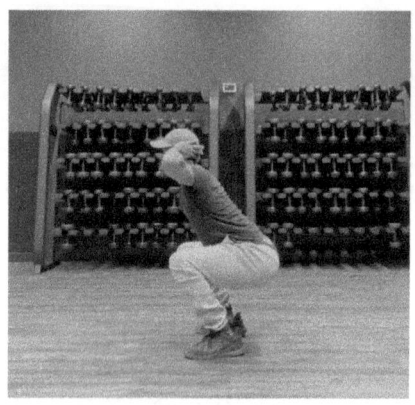

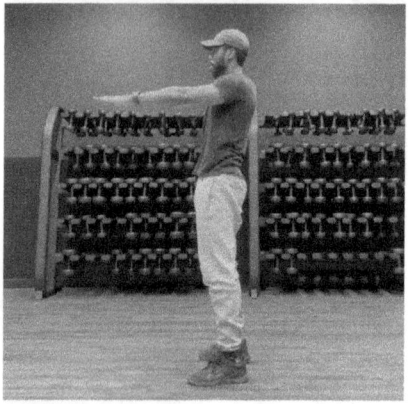

5.) As you're coming back up from the squatting position, exhale through your mouth.

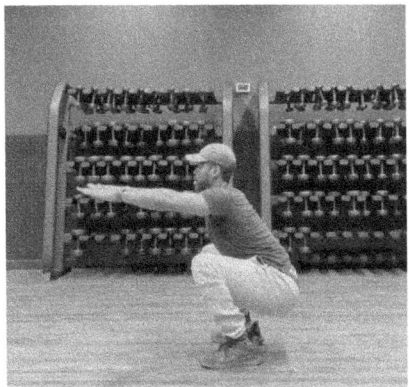

Note: When it comes to hand placement for the standard body weight squat, you can just have them in front of you either both arms straight or elbows bent and hands close to your chest. If you're doing a Prisoner Squat, then you're going to interlock your fingers and place your hands behind your head and perform the squat exercise this way. The key thing to remember is to keep your chest upright. If you notice that while doing the squat exercise this way and your chest dropping towards the ground then change you hand placement.

## Rocket Jumps

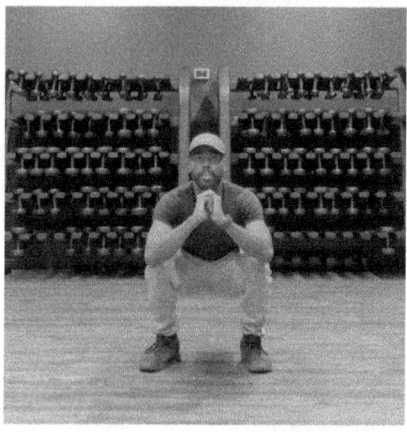

1.) Start in an upright standing position with feet about hip-width apart and hands close to your chest. 2.) Bend at the hips then at the knees, keeping your chest upright and dropping the hips as low as you can. Ideally, you want to get your hips at or below 90 degrees.

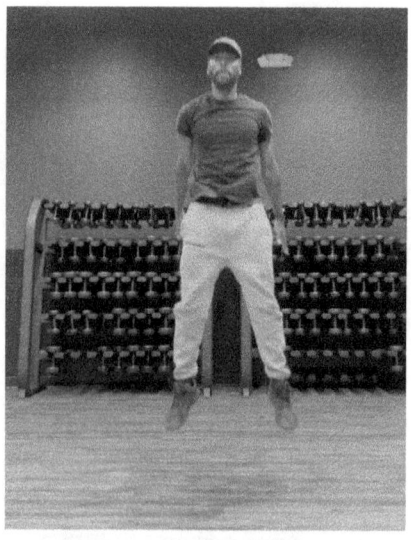

3.) Jump into the air as high as you can. Upon landing, avoid landing directly on your heels. Soften the land with the balls of your feet, drop your hips below 90 degrees, then jump right into the air again.

## Rocket Launchers

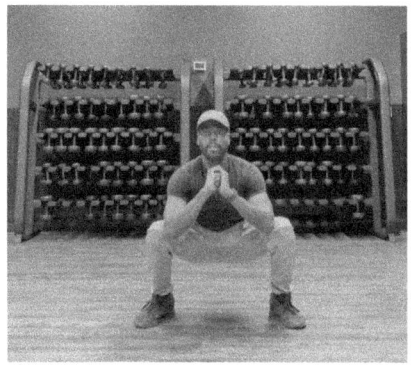

1.) Just like in the Rocket Jump, you're going to start in an upright standing position with feet about hip-width apart and hands close to your chest. 2.) Bend at the hips then at the knees, keeping your chest upright and dropping the hips as low as you can. Ideally you want to get your hips at or below 90 degrees.

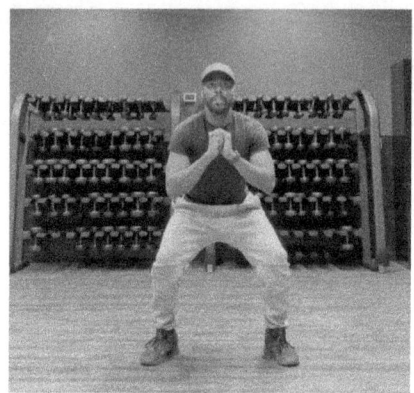

3.) You're going to perform three "pulses" where stay in the squatted position and slightly come above 90 degrees (about 10 degrees) then come back down to 90 degrees (or at least 10 degrees below 90). This is considered a "pulse".

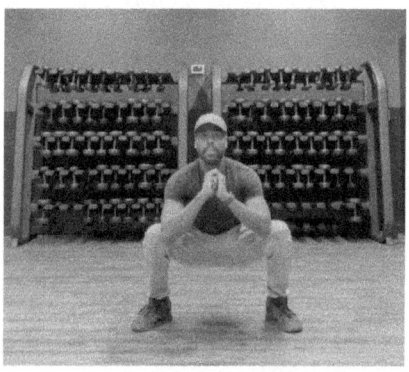

4.) After your third pulse, you're going to drive your arms and jump straight into the air as high as you can.

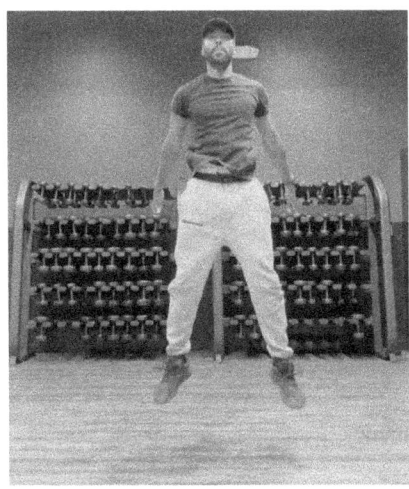

5.) When you land, make sure you implement a soft landing by softening the knees to absorb impact while also preparing you to get right into your next Rocket Launcher.

## Mogul Jump

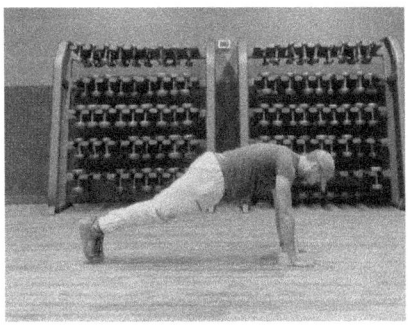

1.) You're going to start on all fours with hands and balls of your feet making contact with the floor. Make sure shoulders are directly over your hands. Both knees are at a 90 degree bend and feet are together.

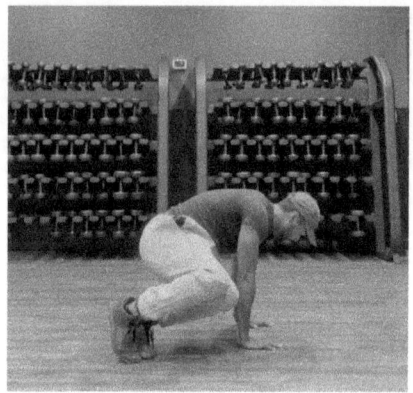

2.) While keeping your arms straight and knees together, you're going to hop and rotate your hips as far as possible to your left side. Make sure your knees don't touch the ground. 3.) Hop a rotate to the right side keeping arms straight and knees together.

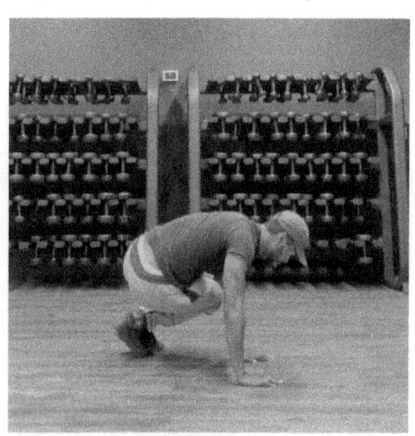

4.) Repeat this movement for time or reps.

## Mountain Climbers

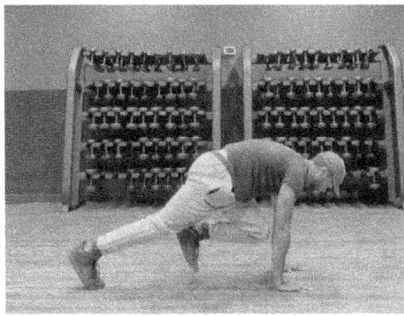

1.) Assume the push-up position with arms straight and both feet together. 2.) Take one leg and drive your knee towards your chest then drive the leg back to starting position.

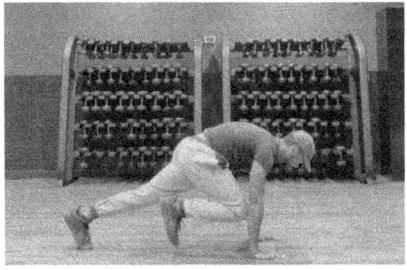

3.) Once foot comes back and ball of feet make contact with the ground, drive your other knee towards your chest. 4.) Repeat this movement either for time duration or reps.

## Mountain Steppers

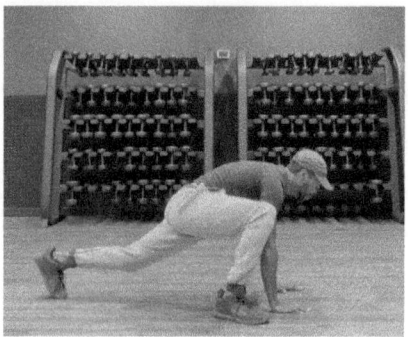

1.) Start in a plank with hands under shoulders.

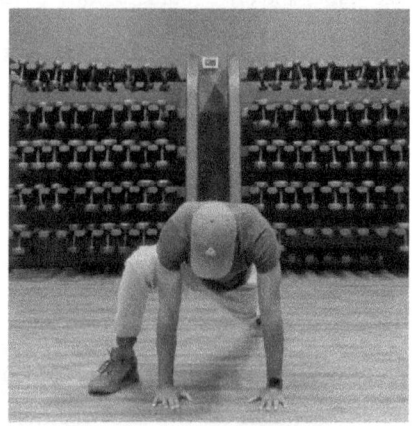

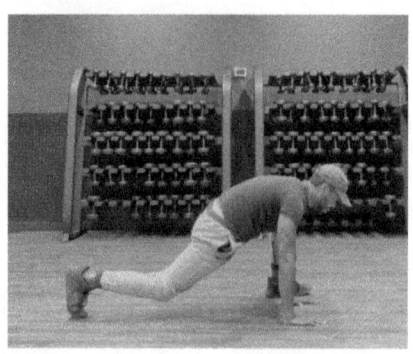

2.) Swing one foot to the outside of your elbows.

# THE FIT BODY F.A.S.T. METHOD 167

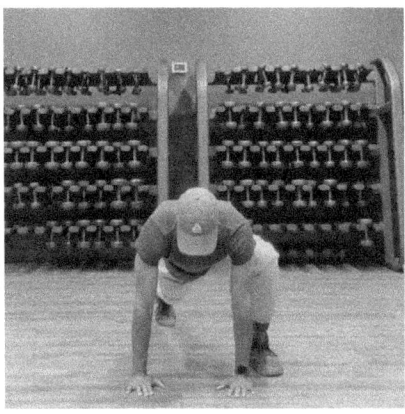

3.) Step it back and switch legs and repeat for reps or time.

## Push Up w/ Shoulder Tap

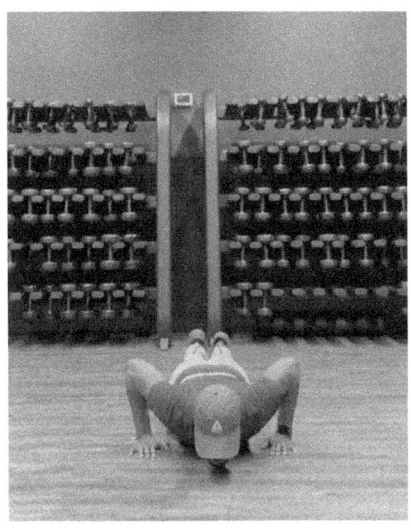

1.) Start with chest on the ground with hands under shoulders.

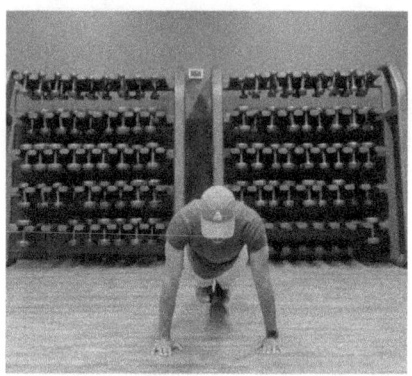

2.) Perform a push-up.

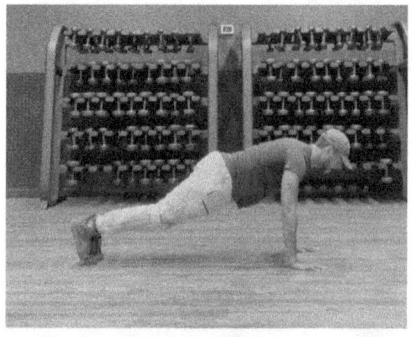

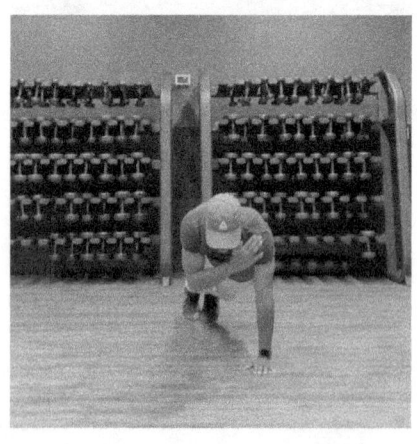

3.) Tap one shoulder with the opposite hand. 4.) Tap the other shoulder, then repeat push up.

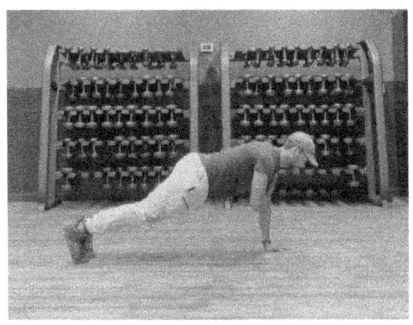

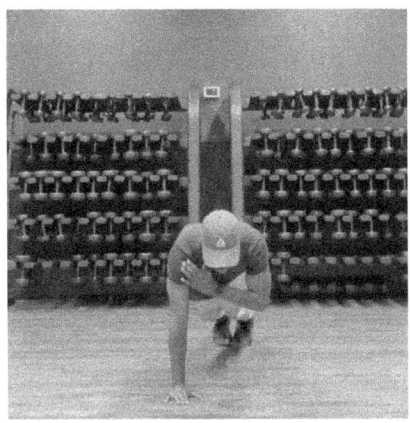

## Dumbbell Exercises

## Weighted Alternating Lunges

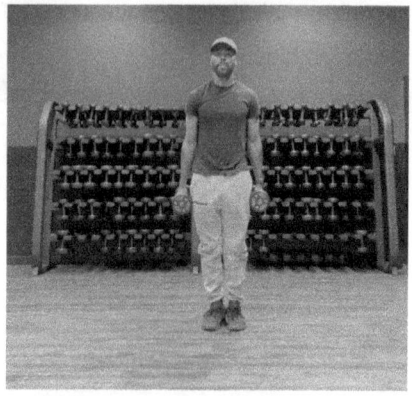

1.) Stand tall holding dumbbells at your sides.

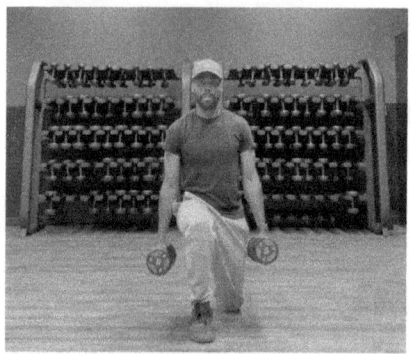

2.) Step one foot forward and bend both knees. Remember to keep heels on the ground for the front foot.

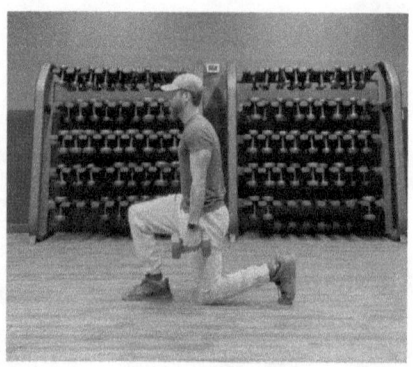

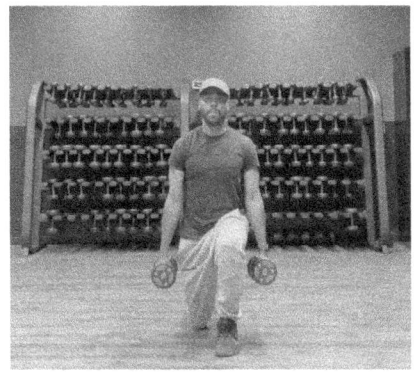

3.) Push through the front foot back to standing position, then step forward with the other foot.

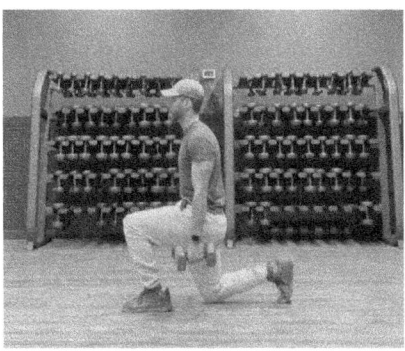

4.) Keep your chest up and repeat.

## Weighted Curtsy Lunges

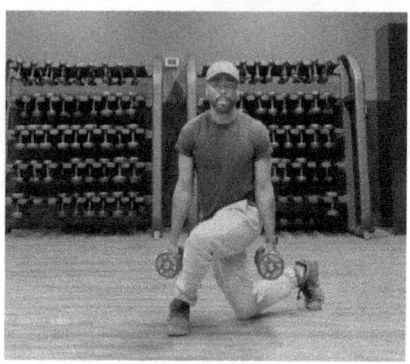

Follow exact same steps at bodyweight curtsy, only this time you're holding weights by your side.

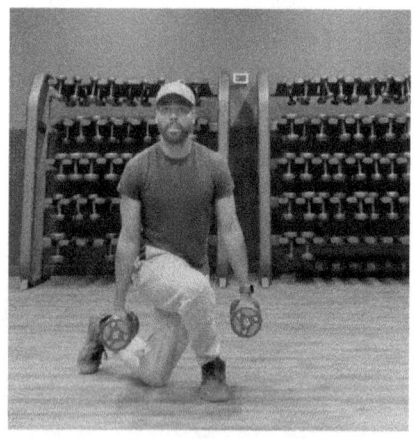

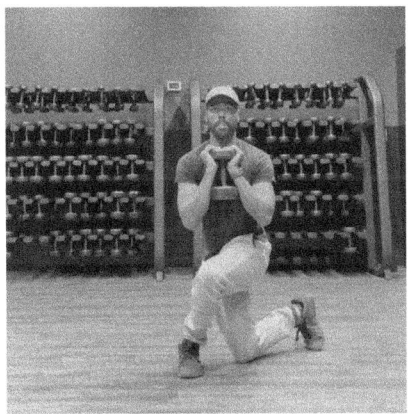

If you are using one dumbbell instead of two, hold the weight in a goblet position, keeping it close to your chest.

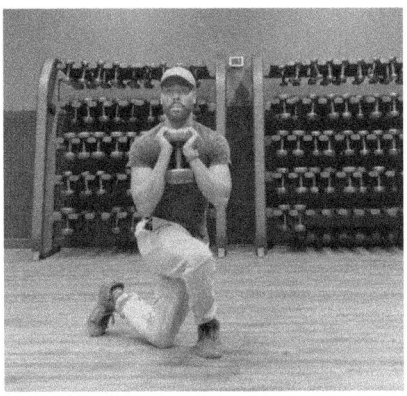

## Lateral Weight Lunges

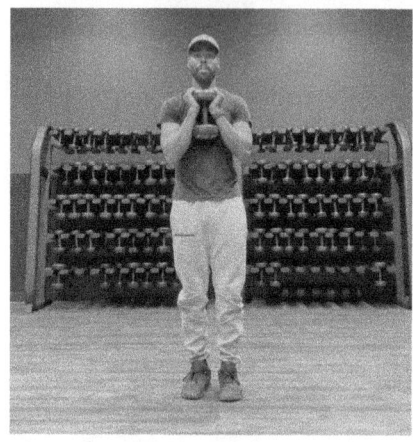

1.) Stand tall holding dumbbells at your sides or if holding only one dumbbell, then keep it close to your chest.

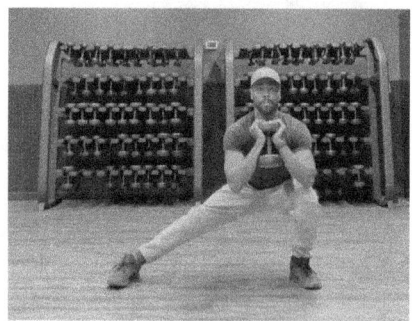

2.) Step one foot out to the side. 3.) Bend the stepping knee and push hips back. 4.) Keep the other leg straight and chest up.

# THE FIT BODY F.A.S.T. METHOD

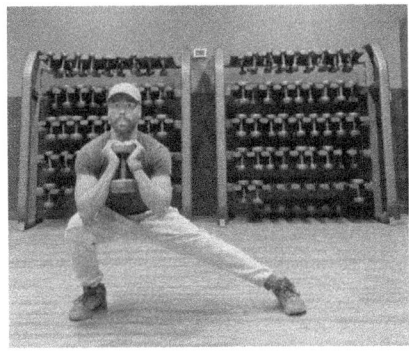

5.) Push off the bent leg to stand, then switch sides.

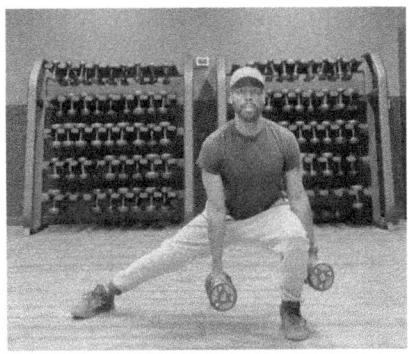

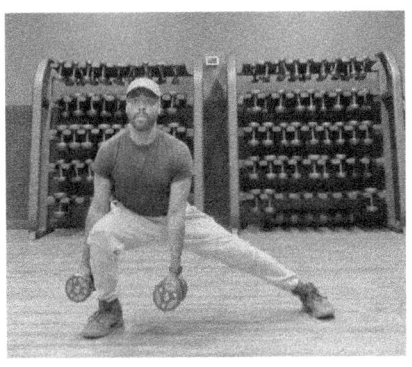

## Weighted Lunge to High Knee

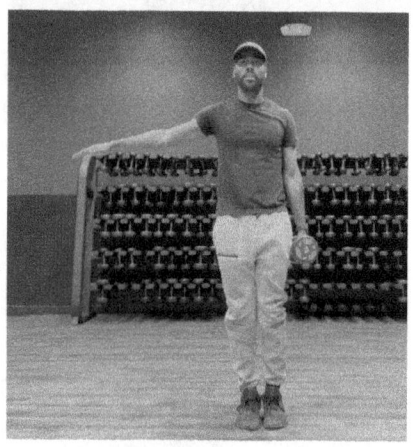

1.) Stand tall holding a dumbbell at your side and opposite arm either extended out on the hip, whichever is comfortable.

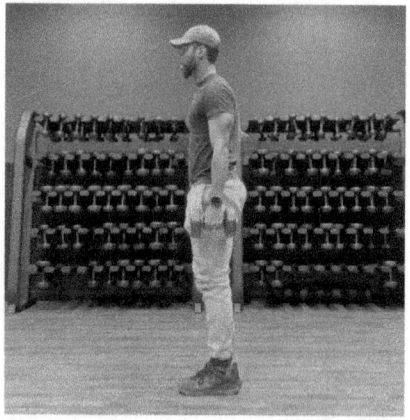

# THE FIT BODY F.A.S.T. METHOD

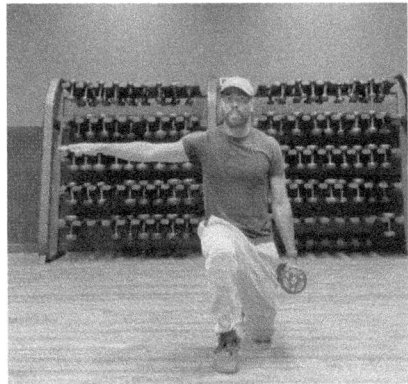

2.) Step one foot forward and bend both knees.

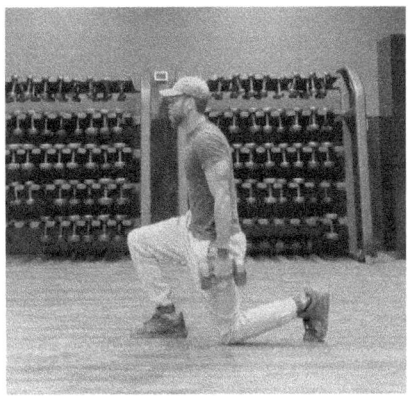

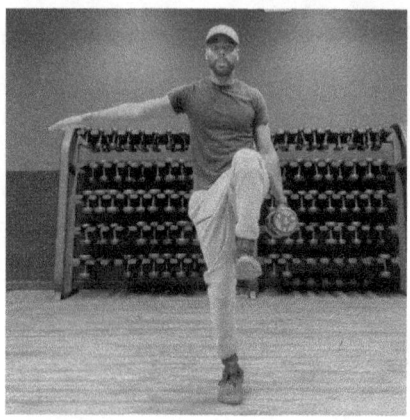

3.) Push through the front foot to stand. 4.) As you stand, lift the back knee up high.

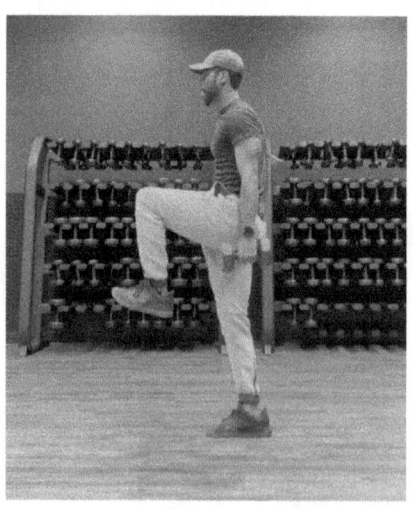

5.) Lower the foot, switch sides, and repeat.

## Dumbbell Goblet Squat

# THE FIT BODY F.A.S.T. METHOD

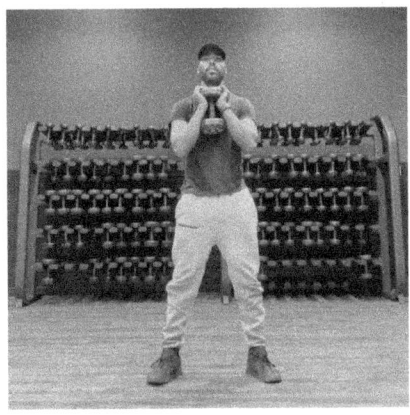

1.) Hold one dumbbell close to your chest with both hands. 2.) Stand with feet a little wider than hips.

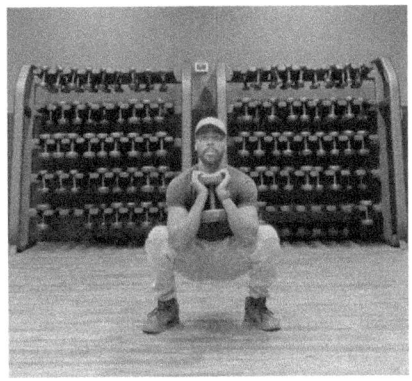

3.) Sit back and bend knees to squat down. 4.) Keep chest up and heels on the floor. 5.) Push through your heels to stand back up.

## Bent Over Row

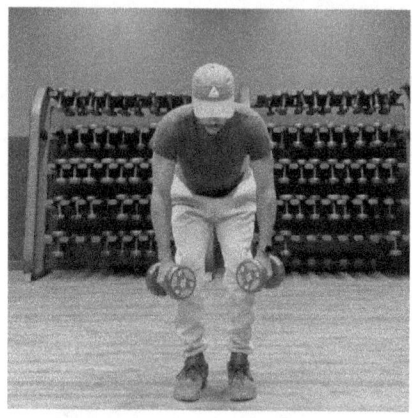

1.) Hold dumbbells down in front of you with palms towards you and bend forward at the hips. 2.) Keep your back flat and knees slightly bent.

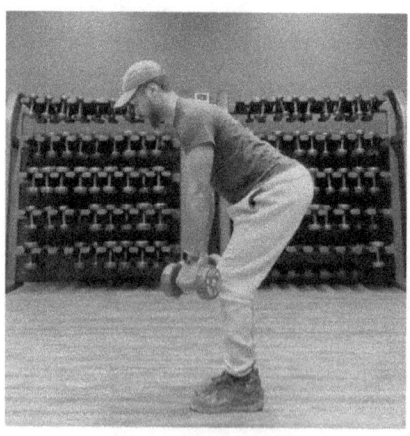

3.) Pull the weights up toward your ribs. 4.) Squeeze your shoulder blades. 5.) Lower the weights slowly and repeat.

# THE FIT BODY F.A.S.T. METHOD

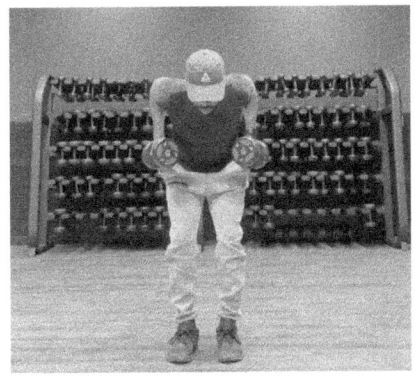

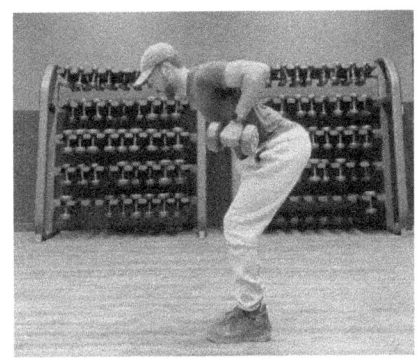

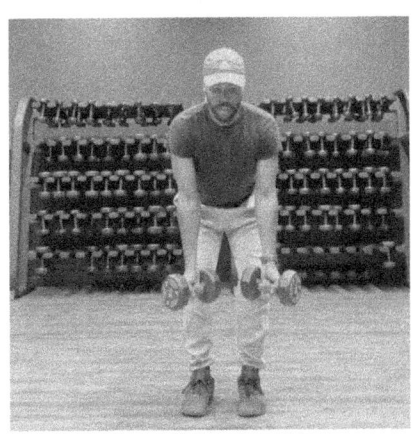

Note: If you're looking to target more bicep, follow the same steps but this time rotate your arms so that your palms are facing forward.

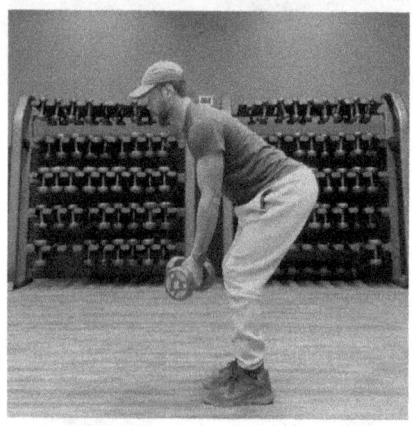

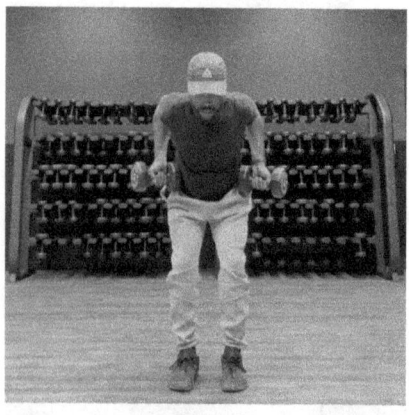

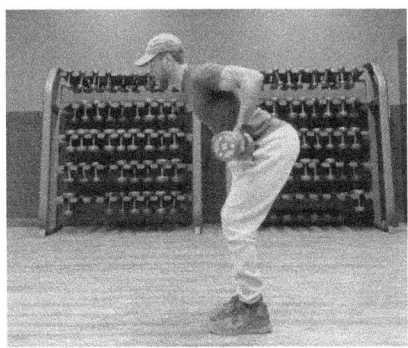

## Dumbbell Romanian Deadlift (RDL)

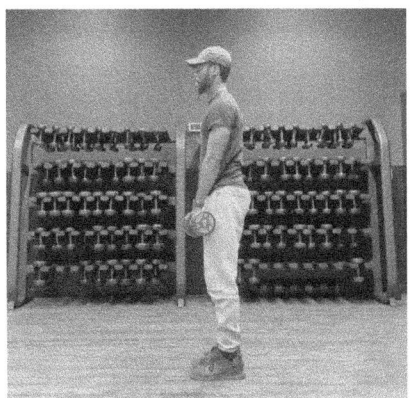

1.) Stand tall holding dumbbells in front of your legs. 2.) Push hips back and lower the weights down your legs. 3.) Keep your back flat and knees slightly bent.

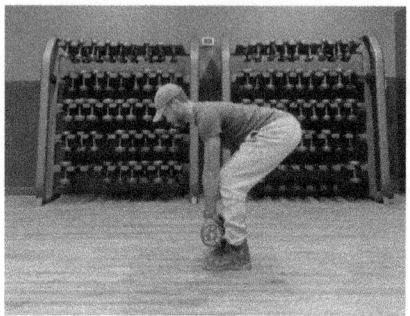

4.) Feel the stretch in your hamstrings and glutes. 5.) Squeeze your glutes and drive hips forward to stand back up.

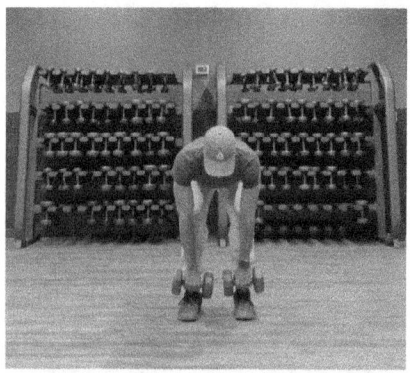

## Dumbbell Thruster

# THE FIT BODY F.A.S.T. METHOD 185

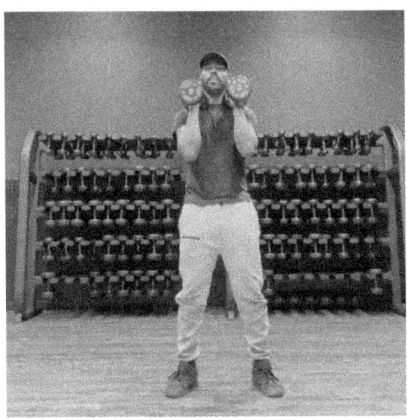

1.) Hold dumbbells at shoulder height. 2.) Squat down by bending knees and hips.

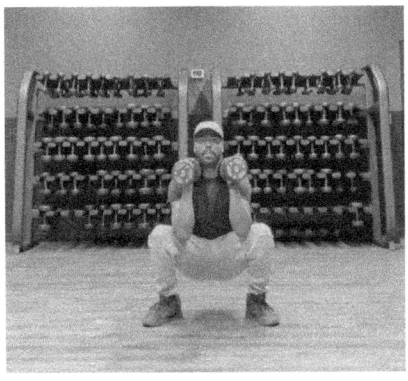

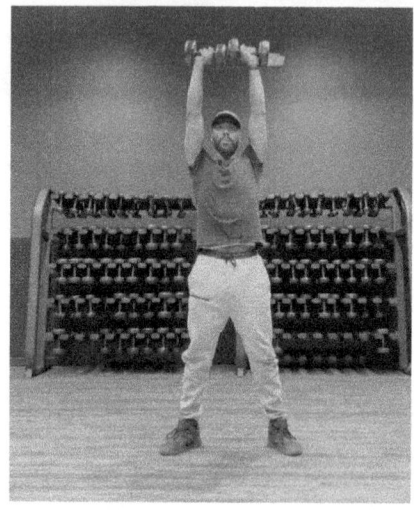

3.) Stand up fast and press the weights overhead. 4.) Lock arms out at the top. 5.) Lower weights back to shoulders and repeat.

## Kettlebell Exercises

## Kettlebell Deadlift

# THE FIT BODY F.A.S.T. METHOD

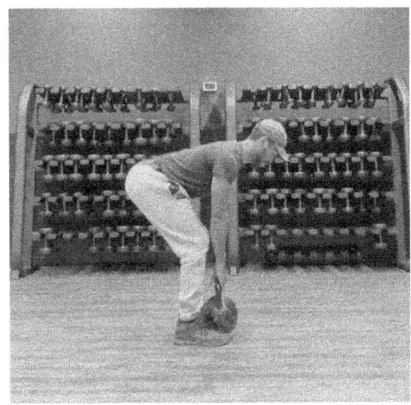

1.) Stand with feet shoulder-width and the kettlebell between your feet. 2.) Push hips back and bend knees to grab the handle. 3.) Keep your back flat and chest up.

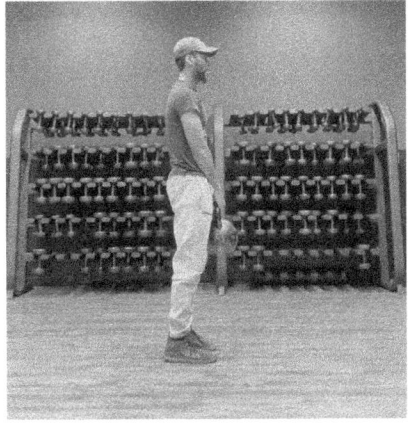

4.) Push through your feet, drive your hips forward, and stand tall. 5.) Lower the kettlebell back down with control.

## Kettlebell Sumo Deadlift

For the Sumo variation, you're going. to follow the same steps as the conventional kettlebell deadlift, however, your stance is going to be wider than hip-width with your toes pointing out about 20 degrees.

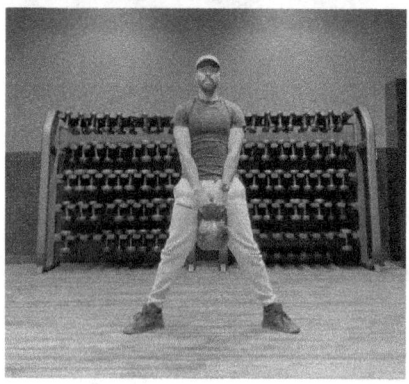

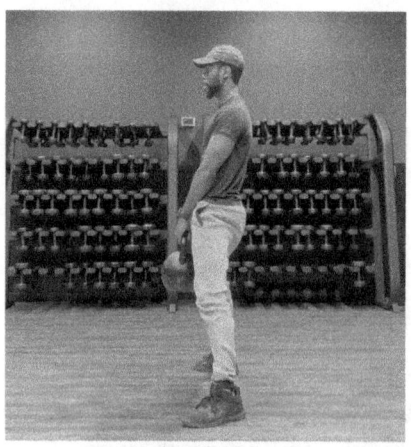

THE FIT BODY F.A.S.T. METHOD 189

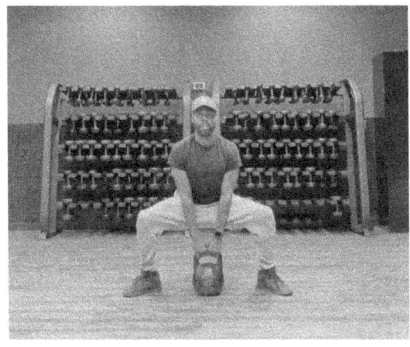

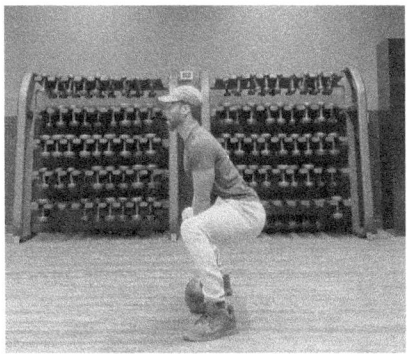

**Kettlebell Single Leg Romanian Deadlift (RDL)**

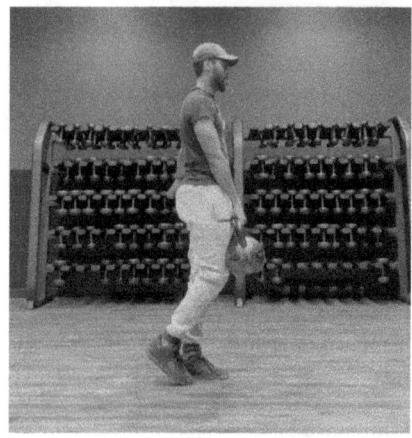

1.) Start in standing position, feet hip-width apart and kettlebell on the ground in between your feet. 2.) Reach down with both hands for the kettlebell, hinging at the hips first, making sure to keep your back straight and shoulders back (Note: If you're looking for more of a challenge, reach for the kettlebell with hand opposite of the working leg). As you're reaching for the bell, you're going to swing your non-working leg behind you, keeping foot flexed and leg straight.

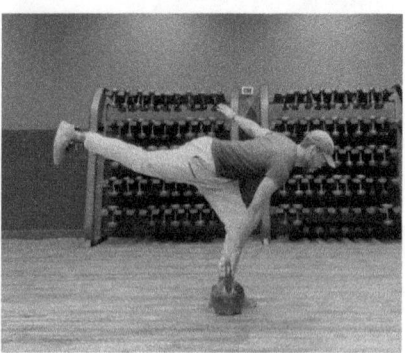

3.) Once you have the kettlebell, squeeze your glutes and drive your hips forward to lift the kettlebell up to standing position. Do not use your arms to lift the kettlebell. They are simply holding the kettlebell. You want your hamstring, back, and glutes to do the lifting. Focus on maintaining a firm grip on the bell and keep arms hanging down the entire movement.

4.) As you're coming up, the non-working leg should swing back down to starting position (think of a pendulum). Make sure to keep shoulders back. 5.) Once at the top, begin to lower the kettlebell back to the floor in the same way you brought it up.

## Kettlebell Kickstand Deadlift

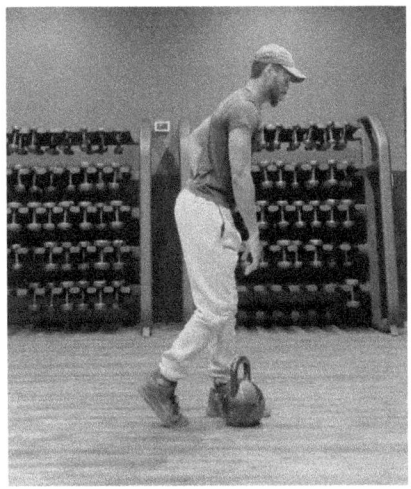

1.) Stand with one foot to the side of the kettlebell and one foot slightly back with your heels elevated so that only the toes touch the floor. 2.) Reach down, keep your back flat and place most of the weight on the front leg.

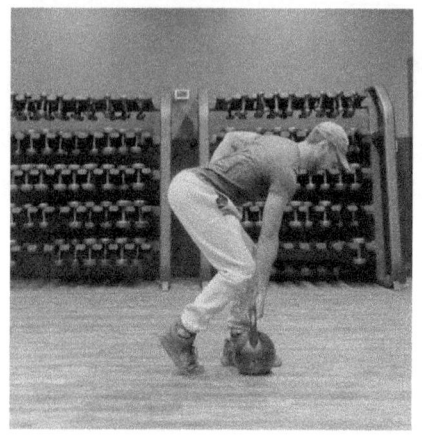

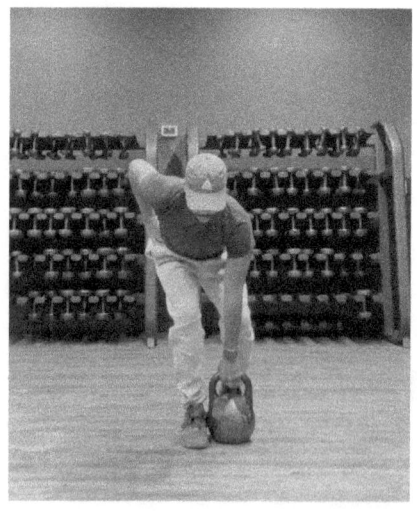

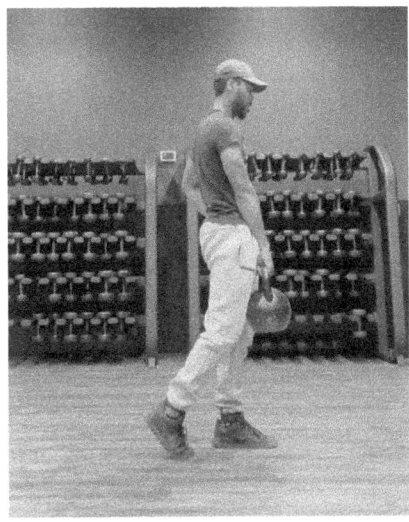

3.) Grab the kettlebell in front of you then squeeze your glutes and drive hips forward to stand up. 4.) Lower the kettlebell by pushing hips back and have a slight bend in the front leg.

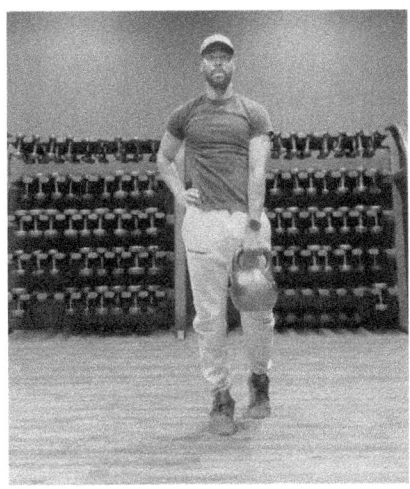

5.) Keep your back flat while still keeping the weight on the front leg. 6.) Bring kettlebell to the ground and repeat.

## Kettlebell Goblet Squat

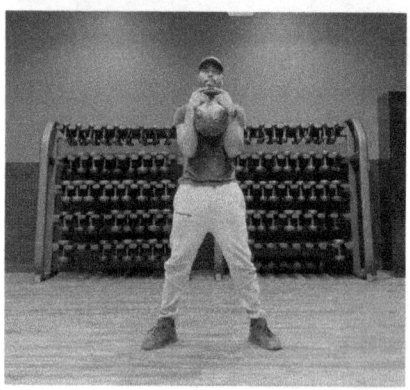

1.) Start by standing with feet a little wider than hip-width apart and toes turned out about 10 degrees. Hold the kettlebell by the horns (the sides of the handle) with both hands while keeping the bell close to your chest and elbows tight against your ribs pointing down. 2.) You're going to squat with the kettlebell close to your chest hingeing at the hips first then bend you knees.

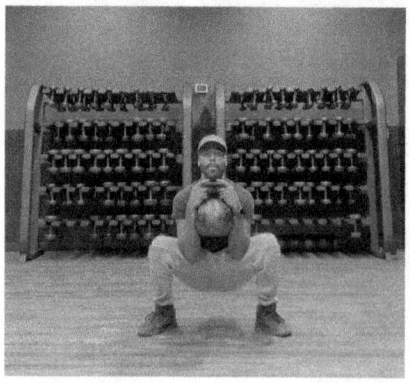

3.) As you squat lower, you'll want to drive your knees out. This will allow you to go deeper in your squat. Try to get your elbows past your knees. 4.) Once you've reached the bottom, push from your heels back up to standing position, squeezing your glutes at the top.

## Two-Handed Kettlebell Swings

Second only to deadlifts, in terms of personal favorites, is this exercise right here! Because the kettlebell swing is a technical exercise, I will explain it in a little more detail than the previous exercises.

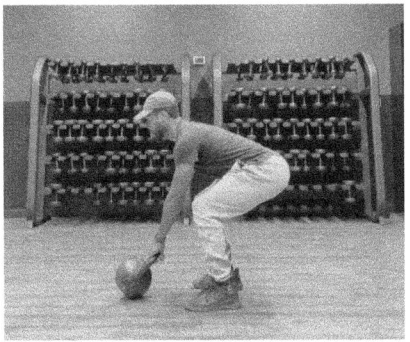

1.) Before you prepare to swing the weight, the kettlebell must start and end on the ground. Therefore for your starting position, the bell isn't going to be in your hands but on the ground in front of you about 6 inches from your toes. 2.) To get started, make sure your feet are about shoulder-width apart with your toes pointing forward.

3.) Lower yourself to the bell, (pushing your hips back and down), keep your shoulders back and down while maintaining neutral spine position from neck to tailbone (make sure to keep in neutral spine throughout entire exercise). Make sure to keep your weight on your heels and establish a two-handed grip on the handle of the bell. (Note:

For single arm swing, you want to grab the kettlebell with your hand placement in the center of the bell.)

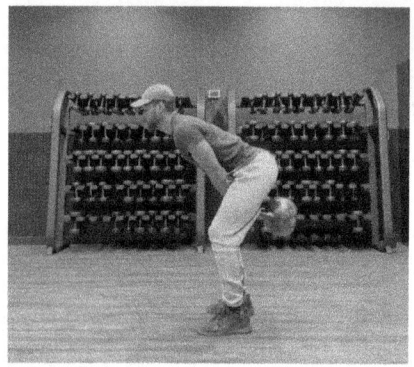

4.) To get some momentum, you're going to perform a back swing from this position first. This means you hike the kettlebell backwards in between your legs before you swing the kettlebell up in front of you. Make sure you're keeping the weight on your heels and your abs and lats are tightened.

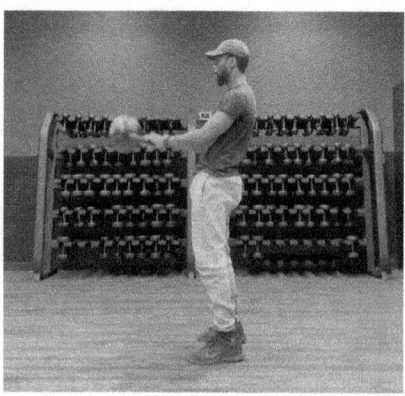

5.) Once the kettlebell is at the peak of the backswing, rapidly drive through your heels, hips and extend your legs into upright standing position while tightening your glutes to perform a powerful pelvic thrust. If done correctly, you should produce enough force to shoot the kettlebell up to hip or chest height. Side note: You should not feel tension in your shoulders. This isn't an upper arm exercise. Your arms should be relaxed, shoulders down and back.

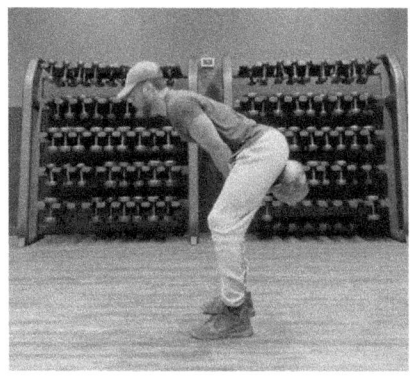

6.) Let gravity take the kettlebell back down and guide it between your legs. Before the kettlebell reaches the inside of your thighs back into the backswing position, make sure you bend at the hips first (as if you're sitting back onto a chair), tighten the abs, and shift weight to your heels. (Reminder: make sure you keep that neutral spine from the head to your tailbone! Try not to tilt your head up or tuck your chin into your chest.)

7.) Once you've reached the peak of your backswing again, proceed with the same pelvic thrust from Step 5. Only this time, because you have some momentum from the first swing, you should be able to swing the kettlebell up to around eye level but try not to go any higher.

8.) Keep swinging momentum until set or round is complete.

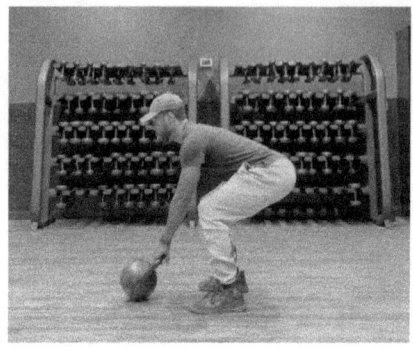

(Note: When putting the kettlebell down after you're done swinging, NEVER stop the momentum of the kettlebell midswing to place it back down. After you finish your last rep, begin to lower your hips back to the ground, as if you're squatting, and shorten your swings. Keep you back straight and shoulders back; DO NOT round your back when putting the kettlebell down at all, otherwise you could suffer lower back injury. Ultimately, you want the kettlebell to end where it began, which is about six inches in front of your feet as in Step 1.

## Core-Focused Exercises

**Back Extensions**

# THE FIT BODY F.A.S.T. METHOD

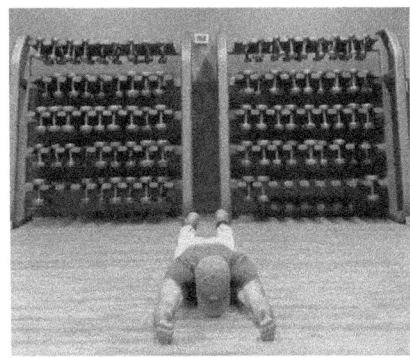

1.) Lie face down on the floor with arms stretched out in front.

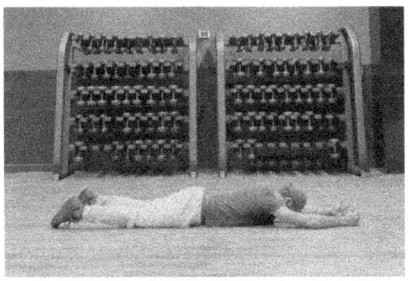

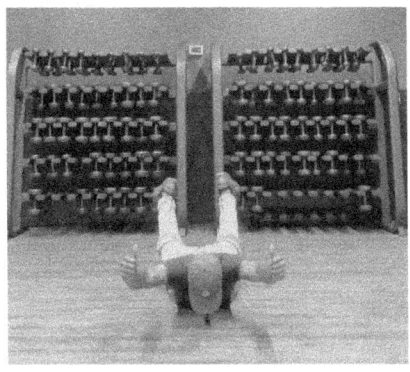

2.) Lift your arms, chest, and legs off the floor at the same time.

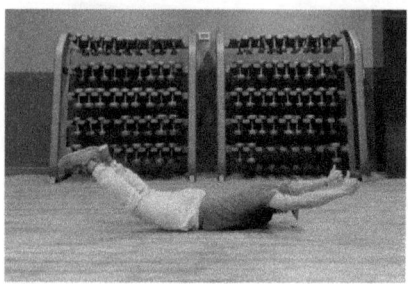

3.) Hold for a moment, keeping your back straight. 4.) Lower back down and repeat.

## Crab Touch

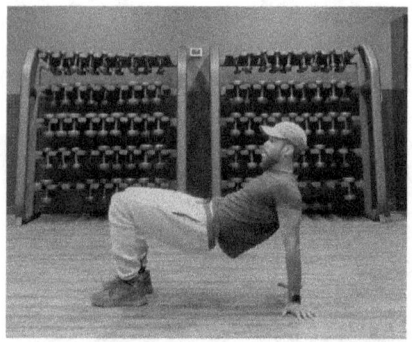

1.) Your going to assume a reverse plank, however knees are bent and feet will be flat on the ground. Remember to keep your hips up off of the ground. 2.) Bend your elbows while lowering your hips but do not let hips touch the ground.

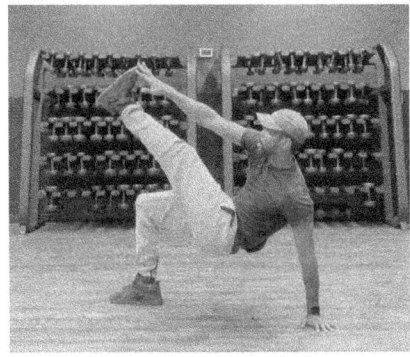

3.) Push through with your arms, straightening them, then kick one leg straight into the air. Drive through with your hips and take your opposite hand and try to touch your toe. 4.) Reset back to starting position and repeat the movement on the opposite side.

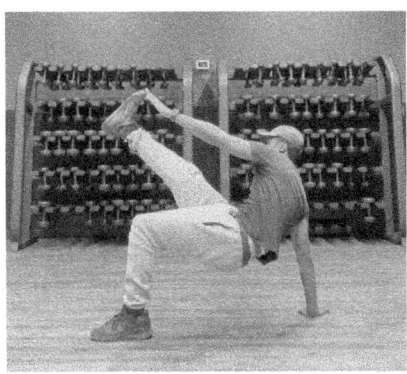

## Reverse Plank

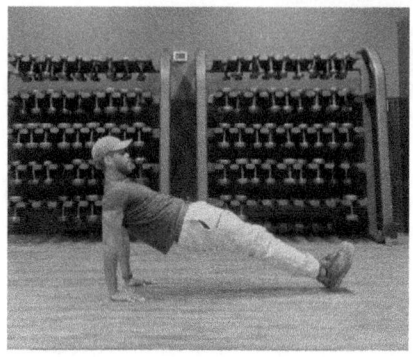

1.) For the reverse plank, you're going to be facing the ceiling with your legs extended forward and arms straight underneath you. 2.) Squeeze your glutes, flex your toes towards the ceiling, and hold this position for time.

## Side Plank

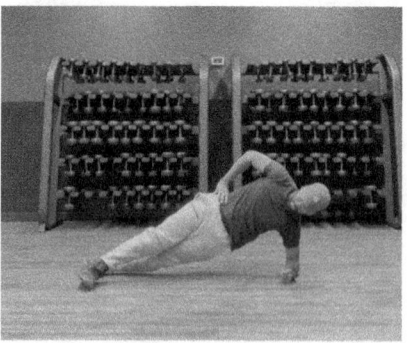

1.) Lie on your side, forearm on the ground, legs straight and feet stacking on one another. The non-working hand will rest on your hip. Raise your hips off the ground and try to keep a straight spine position. Make sure you squeeze your glutes and tighten your stomach. Your

THE FIT BODY F.A.S.T. METHOD 203

feet can either be staggered (one foot in front of the other) or stacked.
2. Hold position for time, then repeat on the other side.

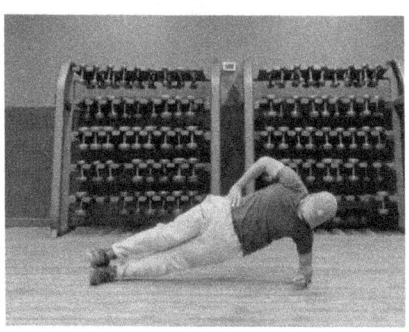

## Plank w/ Side Step

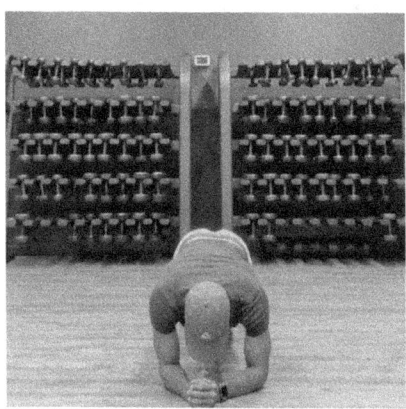

1.) Start in an elbow plank position.

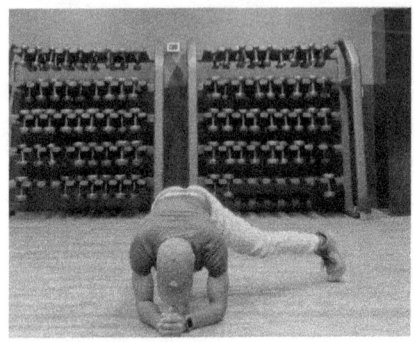

2.) Step one foot out to the side, then back in. 3.) Step the other foot out, then back in. 4.) Keep your body straight and core tight.

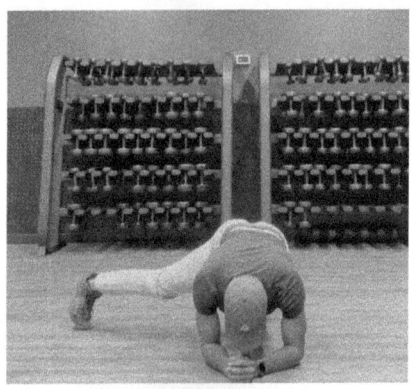

**Side Plank w/ Crunch**

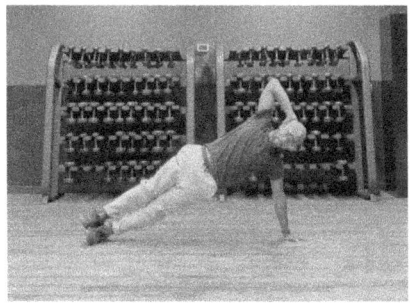

1.) Lie on your side and lift your body into a side plank, supporting yourself with arm extended.

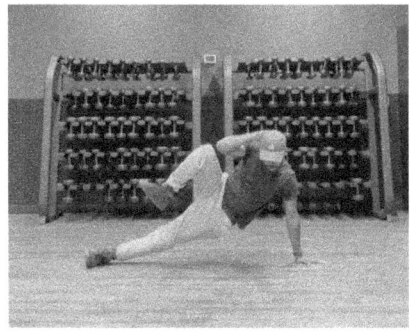

2.) Bring your top knee and elbow toward each other in a crunch.
3.) Straighten back out into the side plank. 4.) Repeat, then switch sides.

## Plank w/ Pull Through

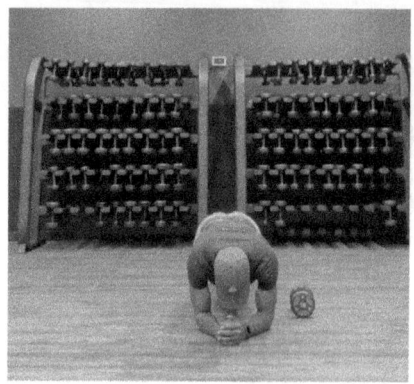

1.) Start in a plank with a dumbbell on the floor beside you.

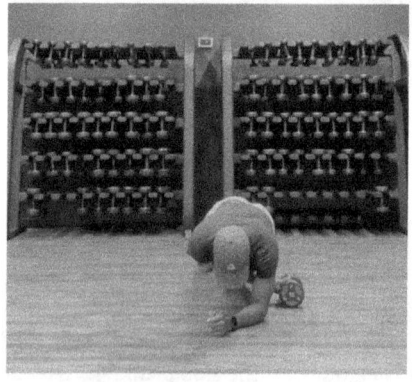

2.) Reach with the opposite hand to pull the dumbbell under your body to the other side.

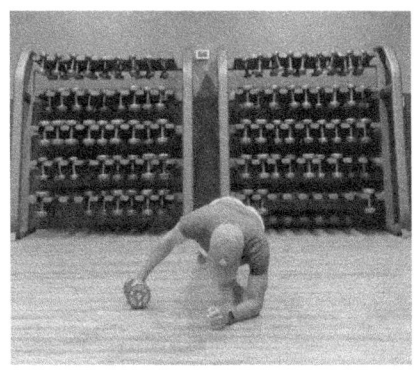

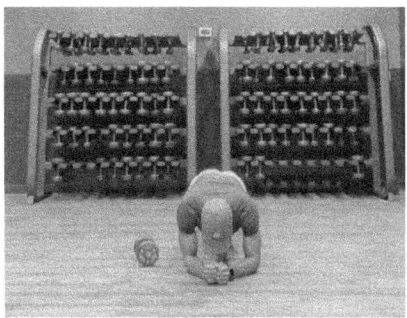

3.) Keep your hips steady, core tight, and bring dumbbell back to the other side.

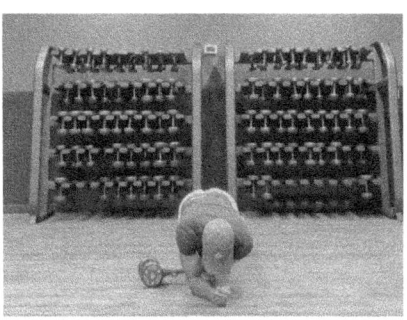

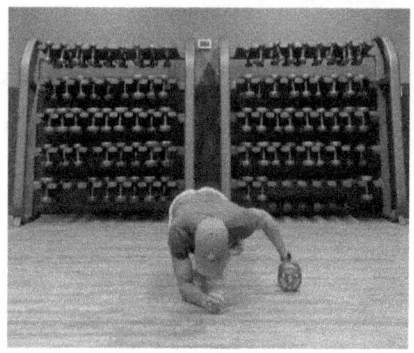

## Renegade Rows

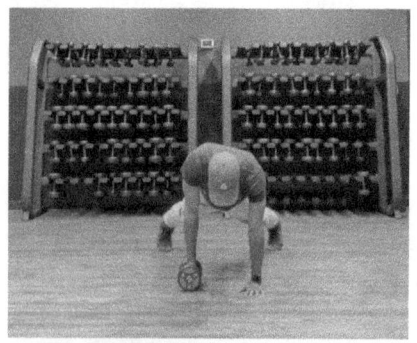

1.) Start in a plank, holding a dumbbell in one hand.

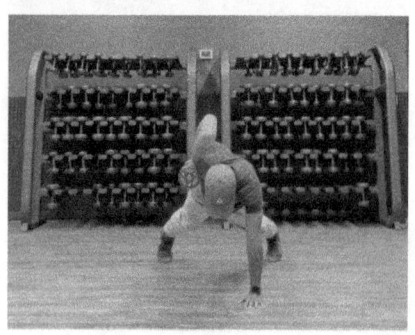

2.) Row one dumbbell up toward your ribs while keeping hips steady.

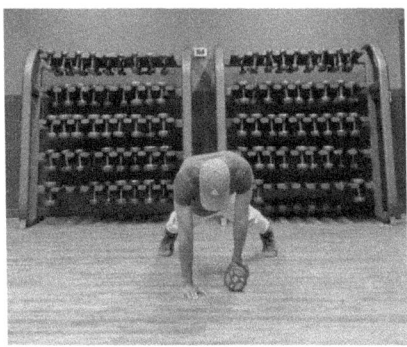

3.) Lower it and pull the dumbbell over to the other side your body.
4.) Perform the row on the opposite side and repeat.

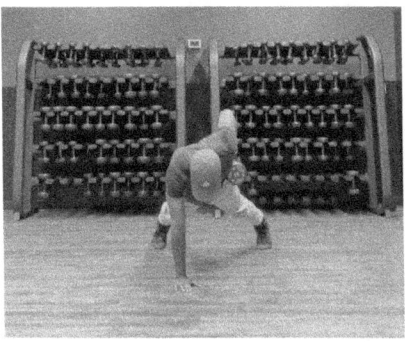

## 1/2 Turkish Get Up (TGU)

Here is another exercise, like the kettlebell swing, that is technical. I will explain this one in more detail as well because, if done correctly, we're talking about major core strengthening benefits from this exercise.

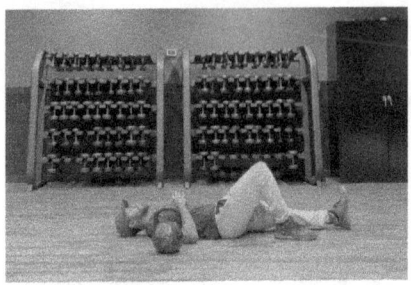

1.) You're going to start off on the floor, laying on your back (supine position) with the kettlebell preferably close to your rib cage or the hip of your dominant hand side. Your legs should start off straight with both of your ankles flexed.

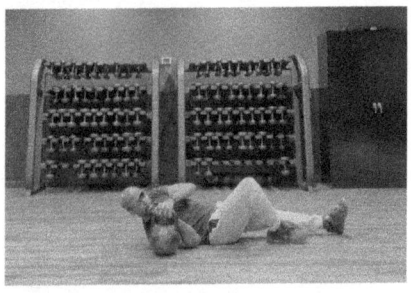

2.) With your dominant hand (the hand closest to the kettlebell) you're going to grip the kettlebell handle, placing the webbing between your thumb and index finger on the corner of the handle, with an underhand grip. Then roll over with your free hand, overhand grip the handle, and assist the working hand in pulling the kettlebell in an upright position over the elbow. (Keep elbow on the ground close to rib cage and keep wrist in straight, locked position)

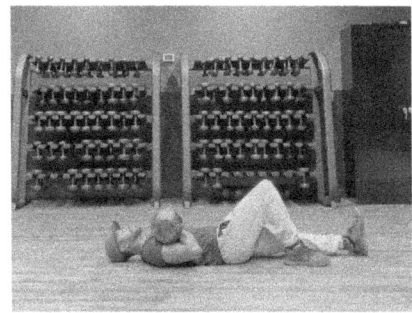

3.) Roll back to supine (laying on your back), then bend the knee and plant the foot (slightly to the outside of the hips) that is on the same side as the kettlebell. Make sure the foot is flat on the ground and your heel is close to your glute. Keep the other leg straight and toes flexed. Rest your free arm on the ground and have elbow about 45° from your rib cage.

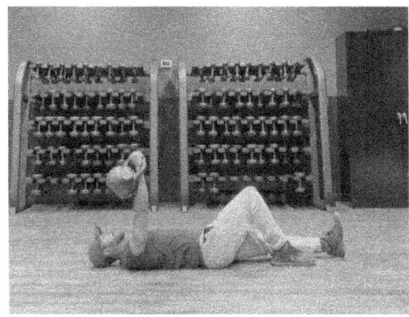

4.) Pack the shoulder joint by pressing your shoulders down and back into the ground, thereby extending the chest. Then press the kettlebell straight into the air making sure to keep the weight directly over the shoulder and not over the face. Keep the wrist locked and don't turn it.

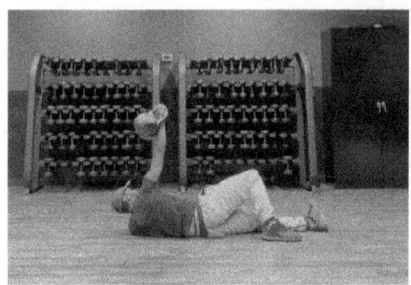

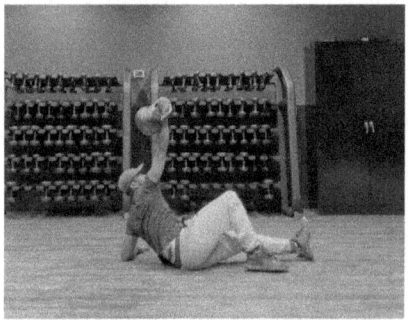

5.) As you're sitting up, you'll transfer the weight of your free arm from the elbow to your forearm, then position your hand to get you in an upright sitting position.

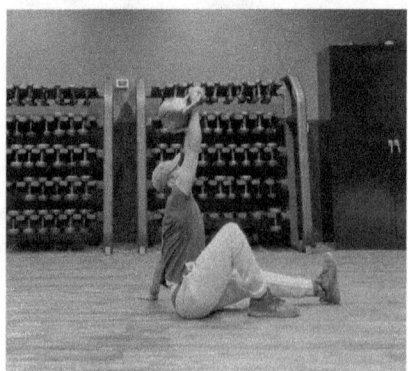

6.) Tighten your abs, then press into the ground with the heel of your planted foot. You're going to rotate to the side of your free arm while sitting up at the same time. Keep the kettlebell straight in the air and in place over the shoulder.

## Deadbug

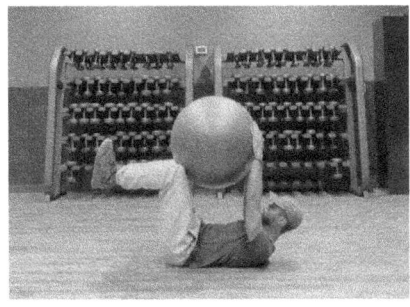

1.) Lie on your back and hold a stability ball between your hands and knees. 2.) Slowly lower one arm and the opposite leg toward the floor.

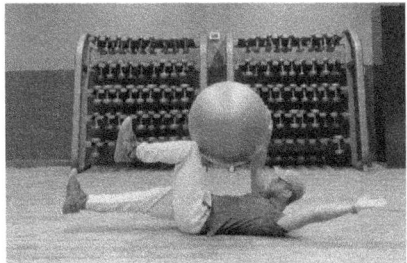

3.) Keep your lower back pressed into the floor. 4.) Bring them back to the center and switch sides and repeat.

## Stability Ball V-Up

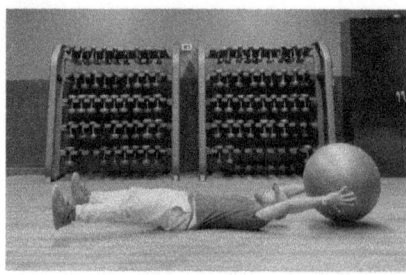

1.) Lie on your back holding a stability ball above your head.

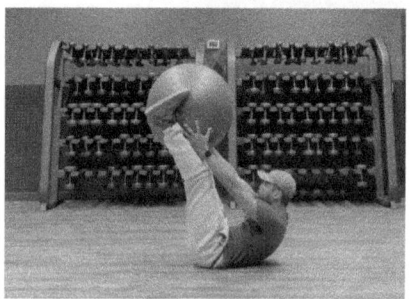

2.) Lift your legs and arms at the same time to meet in the middle.

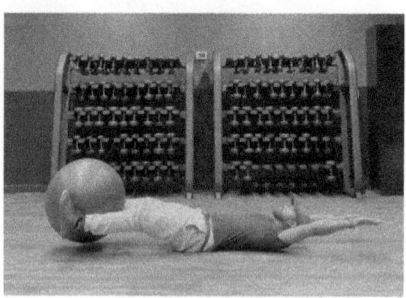

3.) Pass the ball from your hands to your feet.

# THE FIT BODY F.A.S.T. METHOD

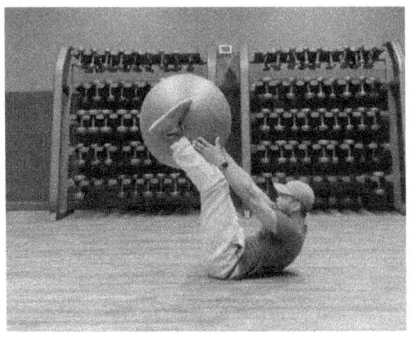

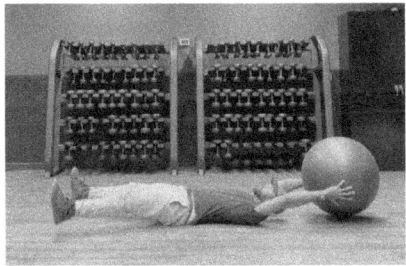

4.) Lower back down and repeat, passing the ball back to your hands.

## Stability Ball Crunch

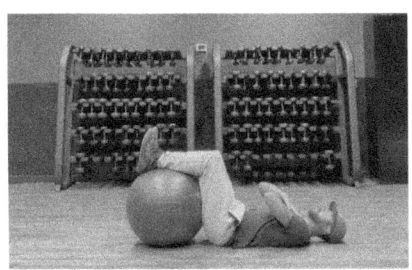

1.) Lie on your back with feet resting on a stability ball. 2.) Place your hands across your chest.

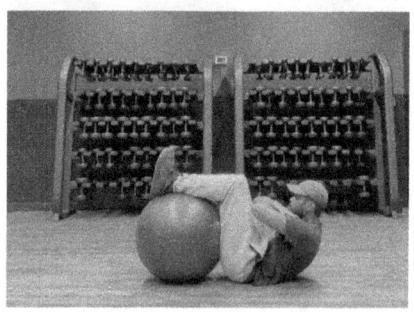

3.) Lift your shoulders off the floor, squeezing your abs and try to get your elbows to touch your knees. 4.) Lower back down slowly and repeat.

## Stability Ball Plank (plus High Plank version)

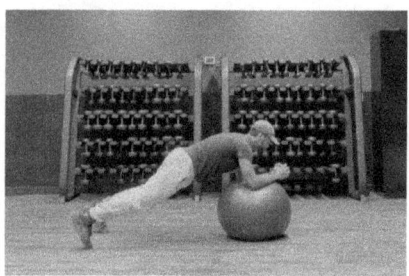

1.) Place your elbows on a stability ball and extend your legs behind you. 2.) Keep your body in a straight line from head to heels.

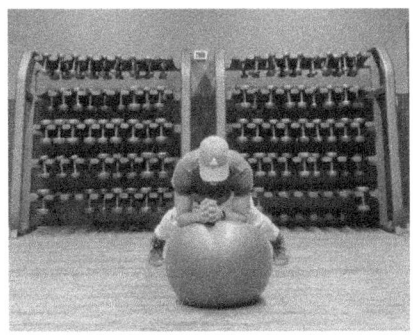

3.) Hold your core tight and stay steady.

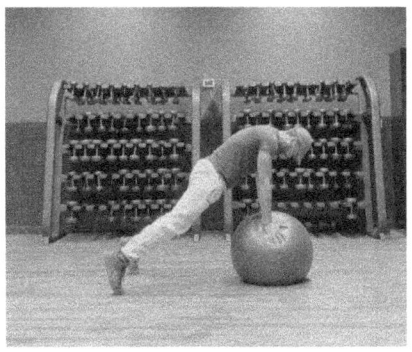

4.) For a high plank, extend your arms and have your hands on the ball with fingers pointing out.

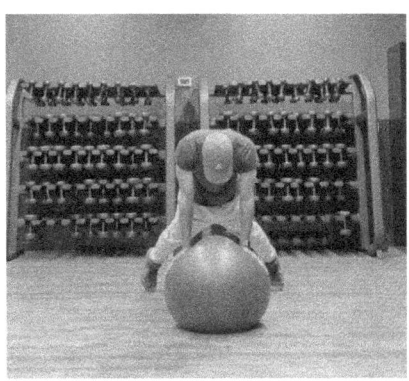

## Stability Ball Ab Rollout (plus Modified version)

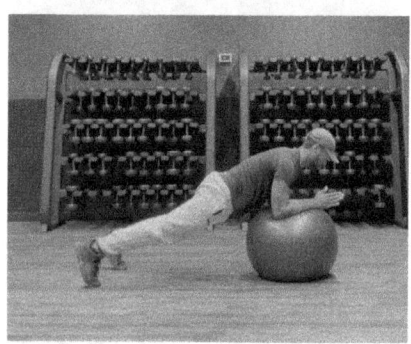

1.) Kneel on the floor with your hands on a stability ball. 2.) Roll the ball forward, extending your body while keeping your core tight.

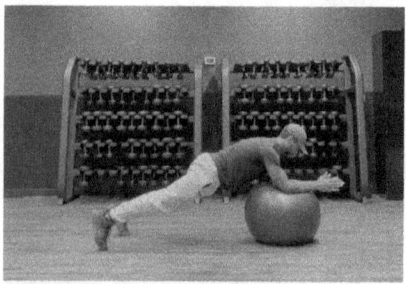

3.) Roll the ball back to start and repeat.

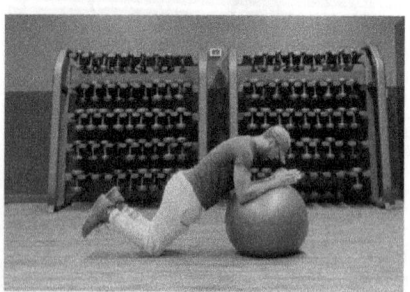

For a modified version, you can have your knees on the ground with feet up.

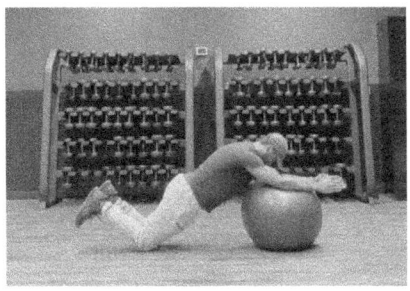

## Stir the Pot

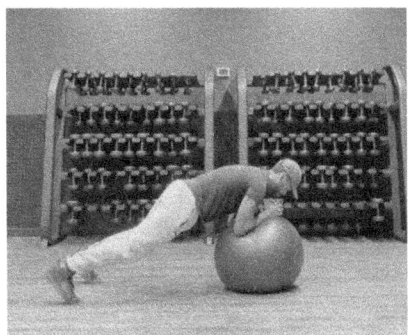

1.) Get into a plank with your elbows on a stability ball. 2.) Make small circles with the ball using your elbows, like stirring a pot.

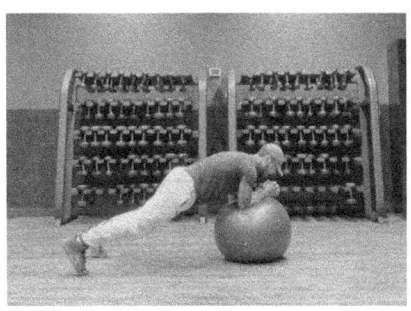

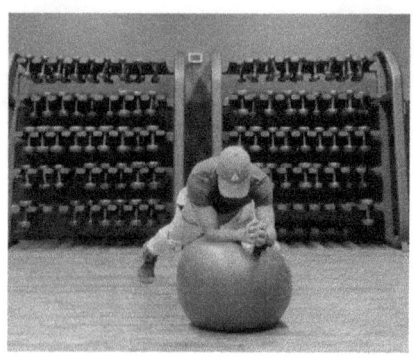

3.) Keep your body straight and core tight. 4.) Switch directions and repeat.

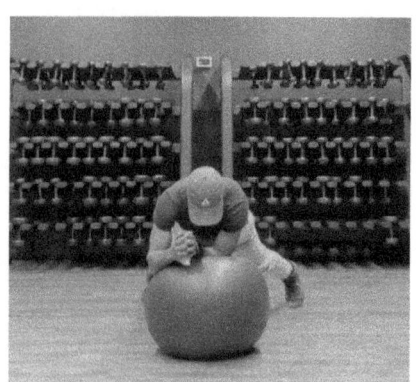

**Stability Ball Tuck & Pike**

# THE FIT BODY F.A.S.T. METHOD

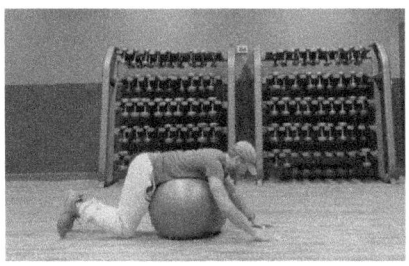

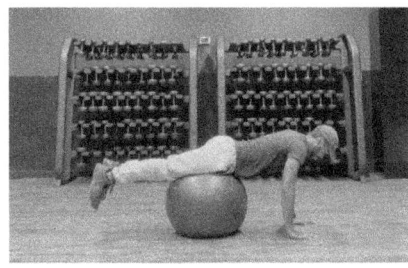

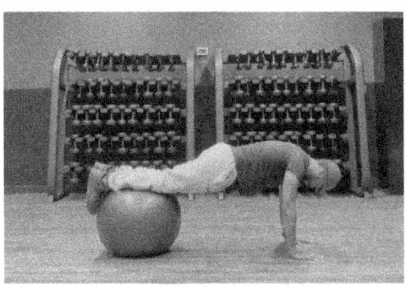

1.) Start in a plank with your shins on a stability ball.

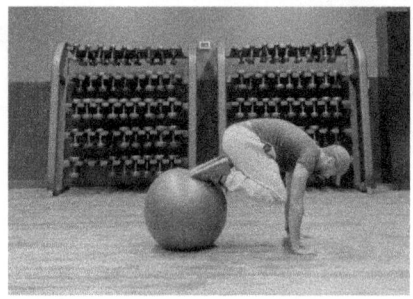

2.) Pull your knees toward your chest (tuck) while rolling the ball forward.

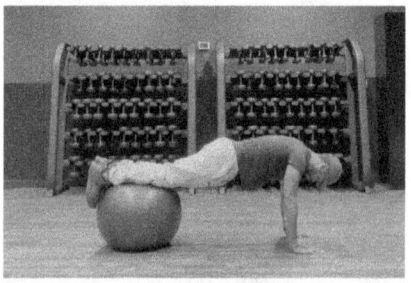

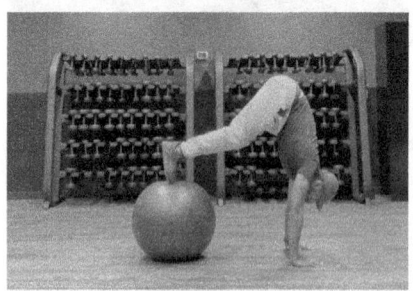

3.) Straighten your legs back to plank, then lift your hips toward the ceiling (pike). 4.) Return to plank and repeat.

## 12-Week Workout Plan (Sample)

### Phase 1 (Weeks 1-4)

#### *Day 1: Squat Focus*

1. Goblet Squats – **4×10**

2. Forward Lunge (DB or BW) – **3×10/leg**

3. Lateral Lunge – **3×10/leg**

4. Bent-Over Row (DB) – **3×12**

5. Stability Ball Plank – **3×30–45 sec**

6. Mountain Steppers – **3×30 sec**

#### *Day 2: Overhead Press Focus*

1. Dumbbell Overhead Press – **4×8–10**

2. Mogul Jump – **3×30 sec**

3. Stability Ball Dead Bug – **3×10/side**

4. Renegade Rows – **3×8/side**

5. Side Plank w/ Step Out – **3×25–30 sec**

### *Day 3: Deadlift Focus*

1. Dumbbell RDL – **4×10**

2. Prisoner Squats – **3×12**

3. Back Extensions – **3×12**

4. Reverse Plank – **3×30 sec**

5. Mountain Climbers – **3×30 sec**

### *Day 4: Chest Press Focus*

1. Floor Press or Push-Ups – **4×8–12**

2. Backward Lunge (DB or BW) – **3×10/leg**

3. Bent-Over Row (DB) – **3×12**

4. Stability Ball Crunch – **3×15**

5. Crab Touch – **3×20 total**

## Phase 2 (Weeks 5-8)

### *Day 1: Squat Focus*

1. Goblet Squat – **5×8**

2. Forward Lunge (DB or BW) – **4×10/leg**

3. Lateral Lunge – **4×8/leg**

4. Bent-Over Row (DB) – **4×10**

5. Stability Ball Plank – **4×30–45 sec**

6. Mountain Steppers – **4×30 sec**

## *Day 2: Overhead Press Focus*

1. Dumbbell Overhead Press – **5×8–10**

2. Mogul Jump – **4×45-sec**

3. Stability Ball Dead Bug – **4×12/side**

4. Renegade Rows – **4×10/side**

5. Side Plank – 4×**30 sec/side**

## *Day 3: Deadlift Focus*

1. Dumbbell RDL – **5×10-12**

2. Prisoner Squats – **4×12**

3. Back Extensions – 4×**12**

4. Reverse Plank – 4×**45 sec**

5. Mountain Climbers – 4×**30 sec**

### *Day 4: Chest Press Focus*

1. Floor Press or Push-Ups – **5×12**

2. Backward Lunge (DB or BW) – **4×10/leg**

3. Bent-Over Row (DB) – **4×12**

4. Stability Ball Crunch – **4×15**

5. Crab Touch – **4×20 total**

## Phase 3 (Weeks 9-12)

### *Day 1: Squat Focus*

1. Back Squat – **5×6**

2. Curtsy Lunge (DB or BW) – **4×10/leg**

3. Kettlebell Goblet Squat – **4×12**

4. Stir the Pot – **4×30 sec**

5. Rocket Jumps – **4×10**

### *Day 2: Overhead Press Focus*

1. Dumbbell Thrusters – **5×12**

2. Lateral Lunges – **4×12/leg**

3. Renegade Rows – **4×12/side**

4. Stability Ball Ab Rollout – **4×45 sec**

5. Mountain Climbers – **4x45 sec**

## *Day 3: Deadlift Focus*

1. Sumo Deadlift – **5×6**

2. Kettlebell RDL – **4×12**

3. Back Extensions – 4×**15**

4. Plank w/ Pull Through – **4×10/side**

5. Kettlebell Swings – **4×25**

## *Day 4: Chest Press Focus*

1. Floor Press or Push-Ups – **5×8–12**

2. Backward Lunge to High Knee Jump (DB or BW) – **4×8-10/leg**

3. Bent-Over Row (DB) – **4×12**

4. Stability Ball V-Up – **4×12**

5. Stability Ball Dead Bug – **4×15/side**

## Simple Workout Formula: How and When to Change Up Your Workout

If you have access to a wide range of equipment, I understand that sometimes you want to experiment with your own workouts or maybe add some of your own exercises to some of the exercises that are in this book. The question I often get from my clients who want to put in the extra work outside of our normal sessions is, "How do I go about adjusting the numbers for my workout?"

Once I figured out what kinds of exercises I feel will work best with my clients, I'd like to start off at a base. I choose somewhere between 3 to 5 exercises and have them perform 8 to 10 reps of those exercises for 3 sets (note: when I say "reps", I'm talking about repetitions or how many times you do or repeat that exercise/movement). The simple reason for this is that those set and rep ranges are manageable for both beginner and intermediate fitness levels.

If you're trying to find how much weight to start off with for a particular exercise try this test: Pick any weight you think would challenge you and do as many reps as you can at that weight. If you're struggling to get to 6 reps, then it's safe to say that the weight may be on the heavier side. Likewise, if you notice that you're barely getting tired and you find yourself anywhere between 15 and 20 reps, then the weight is probably on the lighter side for you.

The "sweet spot" is the 8 to 12 rep range, which is commonly used for muscle building.To all my ladies reading this, I need you to listen carefully: this doesn't mean that you're going to get "bulky"! This just means this is the optimal range to build muscle so that you can become stronger. When you build lean muscle, it helps to increase your metabolism, which is important for burning fat more efficiently and effectively.

You should start at 8 reps for a particular exercise and then gradually work your way up to 12 reps. If you can get to 12 reps with a particular weight, then the next thing I would do is add a fourth set. When you're able to do 4 sets of an exercise for 12 reps, then increase the weight and drop the reps down to 8.

## Functional Over Fancy

There are literally of exercises you can experiment with, however if you put an emphasis on the fundamental four that we talked about earlier in this chapter, whatever workout regimen you choose will be fine. Try not to get too carried away with having a vast catalog of exercises that your regimen becomes too overwhelming.

You don't need to get fancy in order to get results. When in doubt, choose functional over fancy. The exercises that are in this chapter are just a fraction of the exercises I have my clients do, but I try to work with their current limitations and offer different exercises based on what I see. If you have any physical restrictions or limitations, please go and consult with your Physical Therapist. Fitness levels widely vary from client to client and from person to person, so my advice is to attempt what you think meets your current fitness level and and then go from there.

**Key Takeaways:**

- Diet plus exercise is more effective than exercise alone. Don't rely on exercise to make up for poor dietary choices.

- Strive for at least 30 – 45 minutes of high-intensity exercise or up to 60 minutes of moderate intensity exercise a day.

- Focus on the core four exercises (squats, deadlifts, overhead press, vertical/chest press) in your workouts to build a stronger body, increase metabolism, and improve day-to-day functionality.

- Try not to get too obsessed or too carried away experimenting with a bunch of new exercises. Look for exercises that would closely mimic actions or movements you would use for everyday tasks. Remember: functional over fancy.

In the next chapter, and final step of the F.A.S.T Method, we're going to discuss a few nuances that can help you make small changes in order to overcome plateaus before they become an issue with your program.

\*\*\*

For quick access to resources and additional guidance for the material, scan the QR code:

# References

1. Joseph, Gili et al. "A comparison of diet versus diet + exercise programs for health improvement in middle-aged overweight women." *Women's health (London, England)* vol. 16 (2020): 1745506520932372. doi:10.1177/1745506520932372

2. Batrakoulis, Alexios, *et al.* "Comparative Efficacy of 5 Exercise Types on Cardiometabolic Health in Overweight and Obese Adults: A Systematic Review and Network Meta-Analysis of 81 Randomized Controlled Trials." *Circulation: Cardiovascular Quality and Outcomes*, vol. 15, no. 6, June 2022, p. e008243. *American Heart Association*, https://doi.org/10.1161/CIRCOUTCOMES.121.008243

3. Jayedi A, Soltani S, Emadi A, Zargar M, Najafi A. Aerobic Exercise and Weight Loss in Adults: A Systematic Review and Dose-Response Meta-Analysis. JAMA Netw Open. 2024;7(12):e2452185. doi:10.1001/jamanetworkopen.2024.52185

4. La New, Jacquelyn M, and Katarina T Borer. "Effects of Walking Speed on Total and Regional Body Fat in Healthy Postmenopausal Women." *Nutrients* vol. 14,3 627. 31 Jan. 2022, doi:10.3390/nu14030627

# Chapter Ten

# **Tweak**

"The art of life lies in the constant readjustment of our surroundings."

-Kakuzo Okakura

No matter how solid you think your plan is, eventually you're going to need to change things up. It's like having your car on cruise control on the highway, you may need to turn the steering wheel or change the speed from time to time. What was working in the beginning of your program will need to be adjusted...and that's a good thing!

You don't want to get too comfortable with a routine that you forget to make the proper adjustments and you slowly start to slip into a plateau. The reality is that plateaus will happen, but if you're prepared to adapt before the plateau happens, you'll avoid the mistake most people make that keeps them stuck in the same spot after five years. This is what the step of "tweaking" is about. Now let's look at a few areas where you can make some changes before or if you notice your progress starting to slow down.

## Proper Sleep and Recovery Important for Weight Loss

As a coach, I talk a lot about nutrition, training, consistency, and mindset, but one of the biggest factors for effective and sustainable weight loss that often gets overlooked is: sleep and recovery. When it comes to weight loss, if you're making all the right moves in the gym and the kitchen but still feel stuck, stressed, and chronically tired, the missing piece might very well be your sleep.

When you experience quality sleep, your body regulates appetite, balances hormones, and repairs tissue. Basically, it does everything it needs to in order to find balance and improve fat loss. One study followed a group of adults who were restricted in sleep and those who got adequate rest. Those with poor sleep not only consumed more calories, especially at night, but experienced changes in their hunger and satiety hormones that increased the likelihood of overeating.[1]

When those individuals, who were restricted in sleep, returned to getting adequate rest, their weight stabilized and calorie intake dropped. As a side note, I also would like to make the distinction between getting adequate, restful sleep and just getting "regular" sleep. Just because you sleep for 8 hours, doesn't mean it was good quality. Likewise, if you only get 6 hours of sleep, that doesn't mean that the quality of that sleep was terrible. The goal is to not only feel refreshed in the morning but to also give your body enough time throughout the night for proper rest and repair.

In another study that looked at weight loss maintenance, researchers found that those who slept less than six hours per night or had poor sleep quality were more likely to regain a good portion of weight over the next year compared to normal sleepers (those who get the recommended 8 hours of sleep).[2] This just goes to show that sleep quality is more than just feeling refreshed the next day. Sleep quality is also a predictor of whether the weight stays off or if it comes back.

If you are experiencing poor quality sleep and you need make some adjustments in this area, here are a few things I would suggest:

1. ***Anchor Your Sleep Time:*** Try to go to bed at the same time every day (including weekends) to establish a consistent circadian rhythm. This helps with hormone regulation, which will suppress the need to consume extra calories right before bed.

2. ***Tech Wind-down:*** Have ever gone to bed at a reasonable time only to doomscroll and find yourself awake *hours* past your bedtime? To avoid this, you want to try and eliminate screentime at least an hour before bed. There are many built-in tools to help you regulate screentime, but if you need to go the extra mile, set an alarm to remind you before bed. Melatonin, the "sleep hormone", rises naturally at night but it can be disrupted with prolonged blue light stimulation at night.

## What About Fasting?

The next question I naturally get along with nutrition is around the concept of fasting. Personally, I do fast, however I don't do it for weight loss. Sometimes I fast unintentionally due to work and sometimes I do it for other reasons. That said, there are weight loss benefits to fasting when done safely.

Research looking at multiple forms of fasting, has found that intermittent fasting has been shown to assist with weight loss and improve cardiometabolic health.[3] People who fast are able to reduce fat mass and improve insulin sensitivity as well, much like the effects you can expect if you went on a very low-calorie diet.

Prolonged fasting (meaning small periods of fasting done over a long time, not one long, drawn out fast) has also been shown to help improve your body's ability to use or break down fat more efficiently.[4] It was also noted that alternate-day fasting produced greater results than calorie restriction.

Although there are benefits to fasting and many reasons you may want to consider a fast, keep in mind that this is not a primary means of weight loss. It's more of a supplementary component and you should strongly consider consulting with a professional before you decide to go on an unsupervised fast.

## Alcohol's Effect on Weight Loss

I'm always asked about my opinion on alcohol and whether or not it's ok to consume occasionally. This is my response: alcohol provides no value to your weight loss or your health in general, and yes that includes wine.

Alcohol, much like fat, is calorically dense at 7 calories per gram. Unlike fat however, alcohol provides no nutritional or metabolic benefit, so those calories are essentially "empty". The only reason most people think wine gets a pass is because of compounds such as resveratrol and polyphenols, which are known for its antioxidant and anti-inflammatory properties. Research has also shown that resveratrol is able to help with stress, reduce blood pressure, and regulate blood sugar.

Those same compounds are also found in abundance in plant foods such as grapes, berries, and nuts. So, if you can get those same benefits from just consuming the foods themselves, why would you want to dilute the benefits by adding alcohol?

A meta-analysis found that people who consume alcohol consume *more* total calories than those who don't.[5] What this showed was that alcohol consumption actually stimulates appetite, which means you're more likely to eat more food when alcohol is present than when it's not. In another study that analyzed alcohol intake in men, found that increased alcohol intake, regardless of alcohol type, was associated with modest weight gain over a 4-year period.[6] The latter study did mention that weight gain was a risk factor when consumption levels were above "moderation".

Moderation is a tricky word and I try to avoid it as much as possible because moderation literally varies from person to person. We say "everything in moderation" to justify behaviors or things that might not be good for us, and at the same time it shields us from criticism because no person can determine how much of something is "enough" for what a person can or can't handle. Therefore, to be safe, I would rather say use moderation *only* for the things you know are overwhelmingly good and beneficial for you.

In conclusion, if your results aren't progressing as quickly as you think it should, and you're the kind of person who enjoys consuming alcohol regularly (not in an "alcoholic" kind of way but more of an "every weekend" activity) or even occasionally, then my advice to you would be to strongly consider the role you want alcohol to play in regard to your weight loss, stress relief, and your overall health.

## The N.E.A.T Advantage

Lastly, we have a concept most people don't talk about, but could be the slight edge for you in burning extra calories. This is called non-exercise activity thermogenesis (NEAT).

NEAT is the energy you burn throughout the day through movements such as: pacing, walking up the stairs in a building, gardening, standing, and so on. It's basically any movement or activities you perform that isn't considered structured exercise. It's very possible to burn hundreds of calories this way depending on the hobby, level of activity, or movement you're engaged in at the time.

One study showed that individuals who engage in higher levels of NEAT have better insulin sensitivity, lower waist circumference, and improved heart health.[7] You can take advantage of NEAT as well by making small, but intentional "integrations". In other words, find small ways to include more movement or activities within your day without adding more friction. Here are just a few ways to add these integrations if you don't already do them:

1. ***Stand and Move Every Hour***
   If you don't have a watch that already does this, set a timer to remind you to stand, stretch, or walk for at least 2–3 minutes every hour. Break up your sitting time as much as possible.

2. ***Take the Long Route***
   Park farther from your destination or whenever possible, take the stairs instead of elevators or escalators.

3. ***Walk While You Talk***
   When you're on the phone, you can use that as an opportunity to pace around while in conversation. Pacing burns more than sitting.

Remember that tweaks will need to happen no matter how good you think your plan is. These are only just a few common tweaks for you to consider in order to help you break past plateaus and get unstuck. I can't speak for every situation you have that needs to be tweaked but when in doubt, go back to Step 1 (Focus) and go through each step again to see if everything you're doing is bringing you closer to your goal(s).

> **Key Takeaways:**
>
> - To help improve your weight loss and recovery, try to aim for quality, restful sleep and avoid behaviors that negatively affect your sleep such as late screentime and irregular bed times.
>
> - Fasting can be beneficial for weight loss if done correctly and safely.
>
> - Alcohol, including wine, has no benefit to your weight loss and is generally more harmful than helpful.
>
> - Non-exercise activity thermogenesis (NEAT) can help you burn more calories unexpectedly by engaging in small activities that have you move more throughout the day.

This is it! You now have the principles *and* the process to be able to achieve your fit body goals and escape the weight loss traps that have been keeping you stuck. Now it's time to discuss what comes next if you're still feeling stuck.

\*\*\*

For quick access to resources and additional guidance for the material, scan the QR code:

# References

1. Impact of Insufficient Sleep on Weight Gain – Markwald, Rachel R et al. "Impact of insufficient sleep on total daily energy expenditure, food intake, and weight gain." *Proceedings of the National Academy of Sciences of the United States of America* vol. 110,14 (2013): 5695-700. doi:10.1073/pnas.1216951110

2. Insufficient Sleep Predicts Poor Weight Loss – Bogh, Adrian F et al. "Insufficient sleep predicts poor weight loss maintenance after 1 year." *Sleep* vol. 46,5 (2023): zsac295. doi:10.1093/sleep/zsac295

3. Krista A. Varady, Sofia Cienfuegos, Mark Ezpeleta, Kelsey Gabel. 2021. Cardiometabolic Benefits of Intermittent Fasting. *Annual Review Nutrition*. 41:333-361.

4. Gabel, Kelsey et al. "Differential Effects of Alternate-Day Fasting Versus Daily Calorie Restriction on Insulin Resistance." *Obesity (Silver Spring, Md.)* vol. 27,9 (2019): 1443-1450. doi:10.1002/oby.22564

5. Kwok, Alastair et al. "Effect of Alcohol Consumption on Food Energy Intake: A Systematic Review and Meta-Analysis." *British Journal of Nutrition* 121.5 (2019): 481–495. Web.

6. Downer, Mary Kathryn et al. "Change in Alcohol Intake in Relation to Weight Change in a Cohort of US Men with 24 Years of Follow-Up." *Obesity (Silver Spring, Md.)* vol. 25,11 (2017): 1988-1996. doi:10.1002/oby.21979

7. Hamasaki, H., Yanai, H., Mishima, S. *et al.* Correlations of non-exercise activity thermogenesis to metabolic parameters in Japanese patients with type 2 diabetes. *Diabetol Metab Syndr* 5, 26 (2013). https://doi.org/10.1186/1758-5996-5-26

## Chapter Eleven
# Your Next Move...

"Two roads diverged in a wood, and I—I took the one
less traveled by, and that has made all the difference."
-Robert Frost

Although this wasn't a book I intended for you to read all the way through, I am still excited for you if you've made it this far! Hopefully, you've been implementing what you've learned and accessing the extra resources as you were reading. If you've read through this book but haven't done anything yet, and you find yourself still struggling to reach your health and fitness goals, the good news is that you still have a decision to make. As I see it, you have three options.

First, you could go back to what you know. You could go back to following the same strict diets, search for new supplements, and do the same workout routines until you eventually get tired and decide to quit. Second, you could close up this book and do absolutely nothing. You could stay exactly where you are and believe that nothing will work for you, no matter what you do. Or third, you could give this program an honest try for 90 days, do something different, and see where this could take you.

Decide now, out of those three options, which path would be easier for you to take? The last thing I would want for you is go this entire book only to procrastinate and not take any action. Even worse, I would hate for you to stay stuck where you are, doing the same things, and experiencing the same frustrations and struggles, for the next five to ten years. Part of the reason why I wrote this book in the first place was because I wanted to help the people in my life, both personally and professionally, who kept walking down the familiar path of struggle, frustration, and confusion for years.

I wanted this book to cut through noise so that they could finally take control of their weight and their health. That's also my goal for you. By having this book in your hands, you have the principles and methods to serve you as a timeless guide regardless if you see new exercises pop up on your feed each day or if a new diet is being modified each year. I challenge you to go against the popular advice, do something different, and give this program a try. Break the cycle of frustration and give yourself a chance to actually hold onto your results for a lifetime instead of just a short season.

I look forward to see what happens for you in the next three months!

Best of health,

-Marcus

# Frequently Asked Questions

There are things I felt I needed to cover in this book, and many more that I wanted to address but felt it may be too much on the reader. So, this part of the book is meant to tackle some questions you may have had on some subjects that I may have already covered or maybe not covered at all. If you have any question, comment, or concern that wasn't covered here but you would like to bring it to my attention, please feel free to email me at marcus@marcusdennis.com. Thank you!

***

**Q:** What are the BEST exercises I should do to lose weight?

**A:** I teach my clients to aim for full-body workouts, done at moderate to high-intensity, for best results. Do the core four compound movements: squats, deadlifts, chest push/press, and overhead press.

That being said, there is no one particular exercise or group of exercises that beat the tens of thousands that are out there. To be honest, if you preferred not to pick up a weight at all and just followed the "3-2-1 Cardio" method, you could still lose weight! Remember: you can not out train a bad diet. So, even if you had the BEST exercises in your program, you will see little to no results if your diet is lacking.

**Q:** What do you think of Keto?

**A:** I believe the Keto diet has it's short-term benefits, especially when it comes to helping those with epilepsy based on the original research, however, I don't like the idea of Keto for long-term dieting in regards to weight loss. There is no doubt that many people have lost tremendous amounts of weight while on a ketogenic diet, some studied and some anecdotal, but that doesn't negate the overwhelming evidence that a high-fat, low-carb diet comes with many health risks in the long-term. I can't tell you whether you should or shouldn't go on the diet, but I'll put it this way: there's even a vegan version of the Keto diet called the Eco-Atkins Diet...and as clean as that may be, I still don't even support that way of eating.

**Q:** What specific foods should I eat to lose weight quickly?

**A:** First, don't make it a focus to lose weight quickly. If it happens "quickly" from making the right food choices, that's one thing but try not to make that a priority. Second, answering this question in terms of specific foods for you to eat, is out of my scope of practice and should be directed to your Registered Dietician (RD). They're the ones who can legally prescribe/recommend foods to meet your specific needs. All I can say is what I've already mentioned in Chapter 4 and Chapter 8, which is to: 1) include more fiber 2) include more lean protein 3) reduce bad fat intake 4) reduce processed food intake and 5) drink more water. All of these strategies show clear evidence of being positively associated with weight loss. There are many more strategies out there that can work, but I wanted to keep my list short and simple and not overwhelm you.

**Q:** How long will it take for me to lose weight using The Fit Body F.A.S.T Method?

**A:** I have see it take as little as 30 days to start seeing results or it can take as long as a few years if you're not consistent. I would assume that the goal for you is to not only get results fast, but to keep it off long-term. The primary way to do that is by identifying the obstacles that are holding you back, as outlined in Chapter 1, and going through the 4-step plan with an honest effort and an open mind. Results will vary based on where you're starting and how much weight you have to lose, however, you don't want to get caught up in comparing the speed of your success to the speed of someone else's. Trust the process and results will come.

**Q:** How much protein should I be getting?

**A:** It's my belief that most of us in developed countries, especially in the west, should not have to worry about protein intake. Even though numerous studies show that protein intake is positively associated with weight loss, I feel that the 1g of protein/1 lb. of bodyweight equation is a bit much for protein consumption. As a rule of thumb for me, I would recommend between 10 % to 20% of your total calorie intake should be protein, which I feel is more than enough protein.

**Q:** Do you recommend any protein powders or supplements for me to take?

**A:** Although this is a very common question in the health and fitness space, I'm not allowed to make specific recommendations for a particular brand or supplement. Technically, anyone who isn't an RD or nutritionist should not be giving you specific supplement recommendations. However, if you would like to know my thoughts about particular ingredients within a supplement(s) in question, shoot me an email or we could hop on a call and go over them together. I will say that if you are going to choose a particular supplement, then please read the labels to make sure you're not consuming any obvious additives or preservatives than can cause harm to your body. The supplement industry is a multi-billion dollar industry, and I would argue that most companies within the industry do not care about the food you eat, the health risks you currently have, the lifestyle you live, or how their product will affect your health over the long-run. They just want you to buy their product. That being said, I personally opt for plant-based protein supplements to avoid dairy, however I try my best to get mostly everything I need through diet and use protein powders as a last resort depending on the pace of my lifestyle at a given moment.

**Q:** Do carbs make you fat?
**A:** Yes and no. If you consume a fair amount of processed carbs and processed sugar, then the answer is definitely yes! You will have a higher chance of experiencing weight gain from eating those foods. Now, if you're eating carbs in the form of whole foods such as beans, lentils, potatoes, fruits, vegetables, etc., then the answer is NO — these kinds of carbs will not make you fat. In fact, virtually every study that was ever done on regular consumption of fruits and vegetables shows a positive association with weight loss and not weight gain.

**Q:** Can I have alcohol occasionally?

**A:** I talked about alcohol's effect on weight loss in Chapter 10, but as a general rule of thumb, alcohol will always do more harm to the body than good—even if it's wine. Alcohol is associated with unhealthy cravings and weight gain. Aside from what I already shared, there is plenty of other data out there that suggests reasons for why alcohol, even occasional consumption, can damage weight loss efforts. Don't fall for the "moderation" trap. Use the filters I give in this book and decide, "Does drinking this get me closer to my goal or take me further from it?"

**Q:** What's your strategy to recover from soreness after a good workout?

**A:** When it comes to muscle soreness, I prefer and highly recommend percussive therapy (i.e: using a massage gun) but definitely a good stretch is a MUST. Proper recovery also involves getting adequate rest, so make sure you're doing your part to allow ample time for your body to recover and repair after your workout.

# Acknowledgements

This book would not be possible without the support, guidance, and encouragement for everyone who played a major part in my own health & fitness experience, both personally and professionally.

Thank you to my parents, who poured into me to give me a better life so that I can help create a better life for others.

Thank you Theresa for being more than patient with me throughout the course of me writing this book. You understood more than anyone how difficult it was for me to go through this process. I deeply appreciate you doing everything to help make it easier for me to see this project through although there moments where I needed to step away.

Thank you Uncle D for being my mentor and a beacon of encouragement during my low points. You're the one who showed me what was possible within the health & fitness space and it's made all the difference.

Thank you also to my other mentor, Yury Klimovitsky, for allowing me the opportunity to study under you even if it was only for a brief moment. That experience and advice you gave me still sticks with me to this day.

## Special Thanks!

Thank you to my clients, both former and present, for putting your trust in me and allowing me to assist you in your health journey. Your experiences, feedback, and testimonials are what gave me the idea and confidence to write this book. Truly, this book could not have happened without you! By serving you, my sincerest hope is that this work will help to serve others and greatly impact their health journey as well.

To everyone who supported this project well before its official release, I can't thank you enough!

Adam W., Augustine G., Anna C., Caroline M., Christian R., Christina C., Cynthia D., Cynthia W., Ellen W., Gabriella M., Joshua C., Kelly A., Kelly W., Kendra J., Laurie R., Leland C., Lynard C., Marcus D., Michael D., N'Shel D., Nela P., Stephanie D., Susan S.

# About the Author

**Marcus Dennis II, ACE-CHC, CPT** is a Certified Health Coach and Personal Trainer with specialties in Health Behavioral Change, Weight Management and Fitness Nutrition through the American Council on Exercise (ACE). He also serves as a member of the North Carolina Public Health Association (NCPHA) whose mission is to improve public health in the state of North Carolina through education, advocacy, and awareness. He started his health and fitness career back in 2012 and has since worked with well-known fitness franchises, non-profit organizations, and businesses to bring about healthy lifestyle change. For over a decade, Marcus has worked within the fitness industry helping hundreds of clients in areas related to weight loss, fat loss, plant-based nutrition, strength training & conditioning, and athletic performance. Although he was born and raised in Boston, MA, Marcus now resides in Charlotte, North Carolina with his wife and four sons.

www.ingramcontent.com/pod-product-compliance
Lightning Source LLC
Chambersburg PA
CBHW020535030426
42337CB00013B/857